Positive
Colorect

Ordering

Trade bookstores in the U.S. and Canada please contact:

Publishers Group West
1700 Fourth Street, Berkeley CA 94710
Phone: (800) 788-3123   Fax: (510) 528-3444

Hunter House books are available at bulk discounts for textbook course adoptions; to qualifying community, health-care, and government organizations; and for special promotions and fund-raising.
For details please contact:

Special Sales Department
Hunter House Inc., PO Box 2914, Alameda CA 94501-0914
Phone: (510) 865-5282   Fax: (510) 865-4295
E-mail: sales@hunterhouse.com

Individuals can order our books from most bookstores, by calling
(800) 266-5592, or from our website at **www.hunterhouse.com**

Positive Options

for

Colorectal Cancer

Self-Help and Treatment

Carol Ann Larson

Hunter House Inc., Publishers
PO Box 2914
Alameda CA 94501-0914

Library of Congress Cataloging-in-Publication Data

Larson, Carol Ann.
Positive options for colorectal cancer : self-help and treatment / by Carol
Ann Larson.-- 1st ed.   p. cm.
Includes bibliographical references and index.
ISBN 0-89793-446-6
1. Colon (Anatomy)--Cancer--Popular works. 2. Rectum--Cancer--Popular
works. I. Title.
RC280.C6L385 2004
616.99'4347--dc22   2004016124

Project Credits

Cover Design: Brian Dittmar Graphic Design
Illustrations: Rochelle Robbins   Book Production: Hunter House
Copy Editor: Kelley Blewster
Proofreader: John David Marion   Indexer: Nancy D. Peterson
Acquisitions Editor: Jeanne Brondino
Editor: Alexandra Mummery
Publishing Assistant: Antonia T. Lee
Publicist: Jillian Steinberger
Foreign Rights Coordinator: Elisabeth Wohofsky
Customer Service Manager: Christina Sverdrup
Order Fulfillment: Washul Lakdhon
Administrator: Theresa Nelson
Computer Support: Peter Eichelberger
Publisher: Kiran S. Rana

Printed and Bound by Bang Printing, Brainerd, Minnesota

Manufactured in the United States of America

9 8 7 6 5 4 3 2 1   First Edition   05 06 07 08 09

Contents

Foreword

Many of you who have picked up this book have been diagnosed with colon or rectal cancer, know or love someone who has, or live in fear of it because of a family history of the illness. Some of you are interested in maintaining your health in whatever way you can. Others may simply be curious, looking for stories from a patient's point of view that are true and honest. If you fall into one of these groups, you have opened the right book.

Colon and rectal cancer will affect an estimated 147,000 Americans in 2004, with slightly more cases occurring in women than in men. Fifty-seven thousand men and women die of the disease every year, most having lived with their cancer for several years. Yet even in the face of these alarming statistics, a shroud of secrecy surrounds the illness. Despite our culture's ability to openly discuss many subjects once considered taboo, far too many of us feel that to speak of the intestine is somehow improper in polite company.

Carol Larson and the cancer survivors who have contributed their stories to this book are courageous enough to ignore such rules. They face the secrecy head-on and stare it down. They help us to understand the disease and to laugh and cry along with them as they describe their very individual and difficult journeys. Carol's years as an educator serve her well in bringing these stories to us with skill, charm, insight, and humor. I have rarely known anyone who was able to describe with such perceptivity and intelligence her own experience undergoing cancer treatment. Carol and the other survivors' collective experiences—and a lot of very useful medical and scientific information—is presented in this book in a clear and readable fashion.

As a medical oncologist, I have counseled hundreds of patients with colon and rectal cancer as they faced decisions and found their way through today's bewildering medical system. Perhaps more than is the case with most other cancers, up-to-date treatment of colorectal cancer requires a multidisciplinary approach, which means that many different types of medical doctors and professionals are involved at every step of the way. The team may require a general physician, a gastroenterologist, a general surgeon, a surgeon who specializes in colorectal diseases, a medical oncologist, a radiation oncologist, an enterostomal therapist, oncology nurses skilled in delivering chemotherapy, and radiation oncology technicians and nurses. Ms. Larson met with and interviewed professionals from all of these disciplines and more.

Nowadays, with our wealth of online resources, it is easy to find factual information about illness and health. In addition to what can be found on the Internet, a flood of health-related information is available in nearly any hospital or library in the country. However, what is not so easy to come by is the wisdom to put it all together for others who need assistance. *Positive Options for Colorectal Cancer* describes a journey into hostile, foreign territory. It is territory I know well, and one through which I have tried to guide many others. A guidebook is always a useful item to pack on a journey, and here is one of the best.

Kathleen Ogle, M.D.
Medical oncologist

Acknowledgments

This book is a collaborative effort between the members of ACE (Advocates of Colorectal Education) and health-care professionals from the area of Minneapolis/St. Paul, Minnesota.

I wish to express my heartfelt appreciation for the cancer-survivor stories contributed by the following members of ACE: Mary Bakke, Ruth Edstrom, Brenda Elsagher, Marcia Engleson, Jan Gray, Paul Leland, Dan Nosal, Maureen Ness, Jane Nielsen, and Julie Weaver.

Heartfelt gratitude goes to my doctors from the Colon and Rectal Associates Ltd., Dr. Frederic D. Nemer, Dr. Charles O. Finne III, and Dr. Richard E. Karulf as well as to Dr. Amy Thorsen, Dr. Karim Alavi, and Dr. Sharon Dykes, members of the same firm and contributors of medical information in this book. Special thanks go to Cindy Iverson, developmental director of the Minnesota Colon and Rectal Foundation.

Thanks also to Dr. Mark D. Sborov from the Oncology/Hematology Professional Association; Dr. Jan H. Tanghe, gastrologist from Southdale Digestive Diseases, P.A.; Dr. Kathy Ogle, oncologist from the Hennepin County Medical Center; Dr. Gary W. Rene, D.D.S., and the staff of Southdale Dental Associates; Anna Leininger, M.S., certified genetic counselor from the Minnesota Colorectal Cancer Initiative; Alene Christiano, Ed.D.; Vicki Haugen and Julie Powell, enterostomal nurses; Mary Hughes, psychotherapist at Fairview Southdale Hospital; and Jane Nielsen, oncology nurse.

I need to pay tribute to the people who gave me extraordinary support and guidance throughout this project: Donn Poll; Isabella Sartori; Paulette Bates Alden; my writer's group: Rita Benak,

Aimie Klempnauer, Hazel Lutz, Kathy Ogle, and Barb Vaughan; Jane Nielsen and Ruth Edstrom; Dave Larson and Sandy Lyons. I especially thank my brother, Red Lyons, who has encouraged me and so many others to persevere in our writing and to cope with the difficulties of life with a sense of humor.

Special thanks to Jeanne Brondino of Hunter House for your faith in me and for helping me to envision this book, and to my editors, Alexandra Mummery and Kelley Blewster, for your expert craftsmanship and patience.

You have all guided my hand through every chapter and every revision.

I would like to give special credit to my talented illustrator, Rochelle Robbins, who patiently created authentic drawings for this book.

And finally, thanks to the people who were there when I needed them the most: my doctors, nurses, and caregivers; my colleagues from St. Louis Park Schools and from Minnetonka Hennepin County Library; my wonderful friends and extended family of friends; my brother, sister-in-law, sister, nieces, and nephews; my dear departed Aunt Jean; my cousin Meg in California; my husband, Dave, and our three daughters and their families: Tami and Dean Corder, Courtney and Kailey Corder, Laura and Scott Weaver, Abigail Weaver, and Jennifer and Jason Violette. You made my journey with colorectal cancer tolerable and inspired me to do my best.

[The following credits are an extension of the copyright page]
The Advocate newsletter, "Survivor Stories," written by ACE members, all issues, 2002–2004; and excerpt from "Finding Meaning," by Jane Nielsen, Winter 2003. (P. O. 14266, St. Paul MN 55114). Brenda Elsagher interview with Marcia Engleson, *Ostomy Outlook*, newsletter of Minneapolis chapter of the United Ostomy Association, #101, May 2002. Carol Larson, excerpts from "Lessons Learned from Surviving Cancer," *Coping with Cancer*, Nov./Dec. 2001, p. 55. (P. O. Box 682268, Franklin TN 37068). Carol Larson, excerpts from "The Road to Recovery," *Stressfree Living*, Sept. 2003, p. 16. (17483 Sunset Tr., Suite A, Prior Lake MN 55372).

Important Note

The material in this book is intended to provide a review of information regarding colorectal cancer. Every effort has been made to provide accurate and dependable information. The contents of this book have been compiled through professional research and in consultation with medical professionals. However, health-care professionals have differing opinions and advances in medical and scientific research are made very quickly, so some of the information may become outdated.

Therefore, the publisher, authors, and editors, as well as the professionals quoted in the book, cannot be held responsible for any error, omission, or dated material. The authors and publisher assume no responsibility for any outcome of applying the information in this book in a program of self-care or under the care of a licensed practitioner. If you have questions concerning your health or about the application of the information described in this book, consult a qualified health-care professional.

Introduction

If you have been diagnosed with colorectal cancer, you are not alone. Statistics compiled from the American Cancer Society, the American Gastroenterological Association, and the Colon Cancer Alliance indicate the appalling toll on our population taken by this disease. Colorectal cancer (also referred to as colon cancer) has affected too many American lives to be ignored. Here are some statistics:

- Approximately eighty to ninety million Americans are considered at risk for developing colorectal cancer.

- More than 147,000 new cases of colorectal cancer will be diagnosed this year in the United States. That translates into one person diagnosed every four minutes.

- Colorectal cancer is the second-leading cancer-related killer of both men and women in America; it is also the fourth most commonly diagnosed cancer.

- Although the majority of people diagnosed with colorectal cancer are over age fifty, it can strike people of any age, any race.

- Men and women over the age of fifty are at equal risk of developing colorectal cancer.

What's regrettable is that despite these alarming figures—as well as increased information about the importance of early detection—there is an underuse of screening among Americans. This is probably due to social taboos and fear. Colorectal cancer is the disease no one wants to talk about, let alone go in and be tested for. Too many people are reluctant to find out what they need to know about colorectal cancer because they are simply too embarrassed or fearful of what they might find out—but we pay a high price for keeping this secret. The truth is, what you don't know about colorectal cancer could really hurt you, and accurate knowledge about your status could empower you to make good decisions and increase your options for living a healthy life.

As a colorectal cancer patient, I longed for assurances from people who could give me a personal account of their experiences. I wanted firsthand knowledge. To fill this need, three years ago I wrote a book about my journey with colorectal cancer and packed it with information from reliable sources. Still, that wasn't quite enough. I wanted to broaden my base of reference so patients with colorectal cancer could have a more complete picture of what other people had encountered. Writing such a book became my mission.

I soon found a way to accomplish this mission by joining Advocates for Colorectal Education (ACE), a Minnesota-based grassroots nonprofit organization of colorectal cancer survivors. Along with Ruth Edstrom, I became the coeditor of our newsletter, *The Advocate*, which we distributed to all the hospitals in the state. In each issue, survivor stories depicted heartfelt but seldom written-about realities of the ways we coped with our disease. These stories, combined with my own experiences, became an effective way to dramatize technical information. The final product is this book, produced in collaboration with ACE members and medical professionals. In the words of the president of ACE, Jane Nielsen, the fruits of this effort have become a "life-saving legacy for all colorectal cancer patients, their families, and the people who care for them." The stories are all the more powerful for being real and revealing.

The members of our ACE group come from all walks of life, are both men and women, and range in age from thirty to seventy. We have at least one thing in common: We are all too familiar with the ways in which fear can distort the experience of cancer. Most of us started out vowing we would only tell a select few people about our diagnosis. Instead, we've reversed that decision and turned it into a mission to bring our experiences out into the open. We learned invaluable lessons as we struggled to regain our health, and we are convinced it will be beneficial to share them with others.

Positive Options for Colorectal Cancer is a book *for* patients, written *by* patients. It is loaded with practical tips from people who have experienced the problems firsthand. In the book we ask the following questions: What kinds of challenges does a person encounter when first diagnosed with colorectal cancer? What can help when going through invasive tests, negotiating with doctors, and dealing with unfamiliar equipment, drugs, and forms of treatment? How can a person cope with the depressing thoughts that accompany a life-threatening disease? How can people better communicate their needs during a crisis? Does radiation hurt? What things are helpful to consider before surgery? What can help you get through the experience of chemotherapy? What is an ostomy and, if you need one, how does it change your life? What happens to family life and sexuality when cancer strikes and afterward? What is it like to be a cancer survivor?

The technical information contained in this book has been reviewed by the following:

◆ doctors from Colon and Rectal Surgery Associates, Ltd.

◆ oncologists from the Minnesota Oncology/Hematology Professional Association

◆ Anna Leininger, M.S., genetic counselor from the Minnesota Colorectal Cancer Initiative

◆ Jane Nielsen, oncology nurse and president of ACE

◆ Vicki Haugen and Julie Powell, enterostomal nurses from Fairview Hospital, Minneapolis

These health-care professionals were contacted to answer some of the questions we, as patients, wondered about but never asked our doctors when we went through the experience of living day and night with cancer. Some of the information contained in this book is new, such as the effectiveness of "virtual colonoscopy" and the newest findings on genetics and chemotherapy. Progress in treating colorectal cancer will continue; new ways of looking at the disease will develop. What remains the same are the concerns of patients and their families as they find themselves encountering a diagnosis of colorectal cancer.

This is a book for cancer patients, for people who love and care for those patients, and for people just seeking information. It is about exercising positive options to cope with colorectal cancer and to overcome difficulties, and it is about being transformed by the experience.

Survivors

by Ann Favreau, Past President of the United Ostomy Association

Caring people
Conquer affliction
Move as survivors
To comfort others.

Listening ears
Empathetic hearts
Hands outreached
To make a difference.

Touching others
Links of care
Connect us all
In the Healing Circle.

(Reprinted from *The Healing Circle*, available from the United Ostomy Association)

Chapter 1

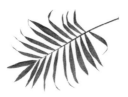

Facing the Unknown

You probably know very little about your colon. Who does? It's like using the plumbing in your house: We rely on it daily, yet most of us don't really know how it works.

Here are the basics: The colon is the large intestine or large bowel (see Figure 1 on page 6). It is approximately three inches in diameter and five feet long. Its job is to absorb water and work like a trash compactor, forming waste matter that can be eliminated through the anus. The beginning of the colon lies just past the ileum. It snakes its way up the right side of the lower abdomen, across, and down the left side, to the sigmoid colon, and then it joins the rectum.

What Is Colorectal Cancer?

Rectal cancers are found in the last six inches of the digestive tract, and colon cancers occur above the rectum, but both rectal and colon cancers are commonly called colorectal cancers. Colorectal cancers develop slowly over the years and most of them begin as *polyps,* flat or grapelike growths that can be detected using either a colonoscope or a sigmoidoscope. Not all polyps are malignant (cancerous). Colorectal cancer can be easily treated in its early stage. If discovered early enough, minor malignancies can be

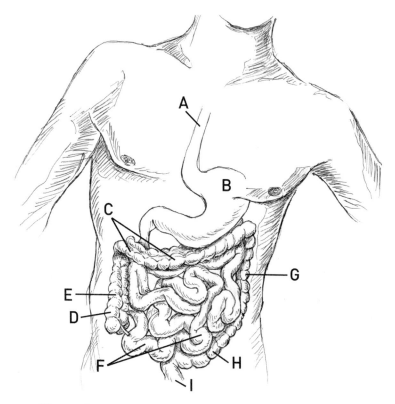

Figure 1. The human digestive tract, including the regions of the large intestine and the small intestine.

A. esophagus	B. stomach
C. transverse colon	D. cecum
E. ascending colon	F. small intestine (ileum)
G. descending colon	H. sigmoid colon I. anus

eliminated during certain tests without further surgery. That's the good news.

The bad news is that a person with colorectal cancer may not have any of the common symptoms, or the signs may be so subtle they go unnoticed. Symptoms can masquerade as other problems, such as ulcers or gastric (stomach) upsets. The only way to be sure is to undergo screening for colorectal cancer.

Warning Signs

The symptoms of colorectal cancer are varied and are easily missed. You may or may not have bleeding, or there may be only traces of blood in your stools. The feeling of general stomach discomfort may be minor.

Symptoms may be related to how far the disease has progressed and the area where the cancer is located. Abdominal cramping and loss of weight, for instance, might be a product of cancer on the right side of the colon (that is, in the portion of the colon on the right side of the torso, also called the *ascending colon*), while problems with constipation and diarrhea might indicate cancer on the left side (also called the *descending colon,* because the contents of the colon are descending toward the rectum and anus). A sense of rectal fullness or a change in the appearance of the stools may signify rectal cancer.

You should not ignore any of the following symptoms:

- ◆ any significant change in bowel habits, such as persistent diarrhea or constipation

- ◆ a narrowing of the stools

- ◆ bleeding

- ◆ abdominal pain that is unexplained

- ◆ bloating

- ◆ fatigue

Paying Attention to Symptoms

When a person is facing an unknown disease, any fear they feel becomes magnified by silence. Some people are so convinced that cancer is a death sentence that they become fatalistic and believe there is nothing they can do. With increasing anxiety, they avoid seeking treatment as long as possible. Other people who experience rectal bleeding attribute it to hemorrhoids. If the bleeding stops, they nervously assume there was no problem and might assume there is no need for further investigation, hoping the problem will go away. These attitudes can just add to the stress level in the long run. Denial can be deadly if it prevents you from getting help.

In my case, the awareness of danger began like a faint siren, hardly noticeable but demanding attention. I was fifty-eight and wondering why I'd been having minor spotting of blood from my rectum for almost a month. The week before a vacation is always grueling, and my job as a high-school teacher in an alternative program was not an easy one, but as much as I tried to tell myself that the physical symptoms, such as spotting, were just "natural," some ancient wisdom inside of me was telling me this was not the case. The blood was bright red, and didn't that mean it wasn't dangerous? Still, I knew it was something I hadn't experienced before, and finally I could make no more excuses.

On my way to a party, I stopped to see a doctor at an urgent-care facility. When he examined me, my worst fears were confirmed. His direct eye contact signaled he was serious about what he was going to say and that there was not going to be an easy fix.

"Any kind of unexplained bleeding is a red flag," he said. "You need to call your doctor right away Monday morning and schedule a colonoscopy. Don't let them lose any time getting you in."

I was stunned. Everything in my life changed. I felt that I had suddenly come up against a barrier and was being directed urgently into unfamiliar territory. It felt like a flashing yellow signal was declaring:

> # DETOUR
> You may have
> colorectal cancer.
> Proceed cautiously.
> Your life may be in danger.

At that moment, without a map, I became sick with fear more than anything else. I felt frustrated and alone, unsure about what I should do. I'd never questioned it before, but now I became aware of my mortality. I knew my health was at risk, and I knew I wanted to survive. I had to face the fact that I might have colorectal cancer, a disease I knew nothing about.

The problem was that no one I knew talked about colorectal cancer, and that made it even more frightening to me. Relatives from both sides of my family had struggled with the disease, but I didn't know what they'd gone through because it was politely hushed up and avoided as a topic of conversation. I wanted to prepare myself for what I was going to have to endure. I needed more information.

I was referred to a gastroenterologist, a doctor who specializes in disorders of the digestive tract, and the following week I went in for a colonoscopy. The doctor found three polyps and removed them immediately. It was lucky for me that he did. The biopsy revealed that two of the polyps were malignant. Though I found out later that the cancer had spread to my lymph nodes, I would probably not be alive today if I had waited longer to go to a doctor.

❡ ❡ ❡

Knowing the early warning signs of colorectal cancer can help a person catch the disease before it has gone too far, as the story below illustrates.

Jane's Story

Jane was in her forties when she noticed subtle, gradual changes in her bowel habits. Like most women she knew, she questioned whether an irregularity was due to something she had eaten or to what is now termed *irritable bowel syndrome*. Those seemed like reasonable explanations to her. But in the back of her mind she wondered if it was something more. She knew colon cancer ran in her family. Her father had been diagnosed with colorectal cancer at the age of sixty-eight. So she kept watching.

Jane also knew from her experience as an oncology nurse that, tragically, many cancers are not caught in time. Many of her patients either discounted their symptoms due to ignorance or fear, or their physicians discounted them. Many went to their deaths consumed with regret for having lacked the courage to speak up or to seek a second opinion.

Jane's awareness paid off. She had a moment of reckoning in the cramped quarters of a hospital employee restroom. She remembers, "I was consumed with pain, holding onto the walls for support, resorting to Lamaze breathing to have a bowel movement. All I could think about was 'What's wrong with this picture?' I couldn't deny it anymore. This was not normal."

At her next OB/GYN physical, she mentioned her periodic difficulty having a bowel movement and the change in her stool's color, texture, and frequency. Since a younger sister had recently undergone gall bladder surgery, the physician ordered an ultrasound and blood work. Later, a reassuring phone call from the doctor's office announced that everything was "okay." Jane was told she was just "a little anemic."

Her search for an accurate diagnosis would have ended there if Jane had not continued it. Physically, she was not convinced that everything was okay. She found a highly regarded general practitioner and asked for help. Without hesitation, the doctor recommended a colonoscopy, because of her symptoms and family history. That intervention changed her life.

As Jane recalls, "The procedure was performed on April Fool's Day. When I was shown the pictures, I knew this was no joke, but something very serious. Following a colon resection for adenocarcinoma (a type of cancer), I received the encouraging news that I was lucky. The cancer had not spread through the intestinal wall or to my lymph nodes. I surrendered eight inches of colon and gained hope the length of a lifetime."

It is possible that working in health care may have given Jane an edge in discovering her cancer in its early stages. But she believes that taking responsibility for knowing her body and reporting her concerns is what really made a difference to her survival.

"We all have instincts," Jane says. "We just have to listen to and honor them with action."

Basic Screening Tests for
Colorectal Cancer

The American Cancer Society has issued the following guidelines for men and women who are over fifty and *not* in a high-risk group for colorectal cancer:

- ◆ an annual fecal occult blood test, in combination with a sigmoidoscopy every five years

- ◆ a barium enema every five years if a colonoscopy is not feasible

- ◆ a colonoscopy every ten years

The screening guidelines for people who *are* in a high-risk group or increased-risk group are determined by the doctor and change depending on the circumstances. A person in a *high-risk group* is someone who has a family history, or known heredity, of colorectal cancer. A person in an *increased-risk group* has one close relative with colorectal cancer before the age of sixty or two close relatives with colorectal cancer at any age.

If there are no known problems, the general guidelines for screening people in high-risk or increased-risk groups are a colonoscopy every three to five years beginning at age forty.

Let's take a look at each of the four tests listed above:

The fecal occult blood test is a chemical (laboratory) test that can detect microscopic evidence of blood in the stool. Usually you take this test by bringing a kit home, obtaining a sample of your stool, and placing it on a treated card. The test is easy to take and relatively inexpensive, but some cancers and polyps may go undetected if they are not bleeding at the time of the test, and some foods or medications may affect the results. To get an accurate reading, your doctor will give you specific instructions on medicinal and dietary restrictions before you take this test.

In the future, colorectal cancers and precancerous tumors may be detected through a similar test that reveals abnormal DNA in stool samples.

*A **sigmoidoscopy*** is a visual examination of the lining of the lower colon and rectum (the last two feet of the intestine). The last part of the colon is S-shaped and is called the *sigmoid colon*. Using a thin, lighted tube called a *flexible sigmoidoscope*, the doctor will examine thirty inches of your lower colon and rectum. By pumping air into the tube, the doctor is also able to see the lining of the colon. The entire test takes less than ten minutes. The air pumped into the tube might cause some minor cramping, not unlike the feeling just before a bowel movement. You might find that deep breathing and relaxation exercises can help you relax to some degree (for one such exercise, see page 18). It can also be helpful to count out the seconds during the most uncomfortable part.

The preparation for a sigmoidoscopy is simpler and less uncomfortable than it is for a colonoscopy. Usually you are required to drink only clear liquids for twelve to twenty-four hours prior and to take two Fleet enemas two hours before the examination. The payoffs of such an exam far outweigh any discomfort you might experience. For people of average risk, the test will reveal up to 70 percent of all polyps in the colon. If anything looks suspicious, the doctor can remove some tissue, biopsy it, and send it to a lab for testing.

The double-contrast barium enema is an X-ray examination of the entire rectum and colon. In this test, barium, a chalklike substance that shows up white on X rays, is usually given as an enema to coat the bowel wall, helping doctors to detect abnormalities that might indicate the presence of colorectal cancer. While taking this test you may experience cramping, like the need to evacuate your bowel, but the test is safe and does not require sedation. The disadvantages of this test are that it detects problems with only a 50 to 80 percent accuracy rate and can only be used for diagnosis. If polyps are discovered, tissue samples must be removed through some other means. This type of test is commonly used as a substitute if a colonoscopy is not possible because of some other problem.

A colonoscopy is the gold standard of colorectal tests. The advantage of a colonoscopy is that it enables the doctor to see the entire colon by inserting a long, flexible tube linked to a video camera and a display unit. The test is usually done on an outpatient basis in a hospital and is performed while the patient is sedated. If a polyp is discovered, it can be painlessly removed right then and there. A sample is then sent to a lab to be examined under a microscope to determine if there is any malignancy. You should be able to get the test results within a few days.

Cleansing of the bowel before a colonoscopy is more involved and complete than it is for other tests. Doctors differ on the kind of preparation they want patients to do for a colonoscopy. Some want their patients to ingest an electrolyte-based solution that is mixed with a gallon of cold water, drinking an eight-ounce glass every ten minutes on the night before the test. One of the common names for this solution is "Go-Lytely," which is a misnomer if there ever was one. You can expect to be running to the bathroom quite often throughout the night before your colonoscopy, which is a good reason for replenishing your fluids the next day. Supposedly, if you drink the Go-Lytely cold, it will taste better. You may request an alternative two-glass version of sodium phosphate, which is much easier to endure, but some doctors prefer the Go-Lytely or something similar for a clearer picture.

Regardless, follow all directions and put discomfort behind you, so to speak, so you can check into the hospital the next morning with your colon fully cleansed. Since most colonoscopies are performed under sedation, the test is usually easier to take than the preparation. The anesthesia, generally injected into your arm, will relax you so that if you do experience some cramping, it will be minor. Since you are being sedated, you will need someone to drive you home after the test.

A colonoscopy is very safe, but there is a slight chance of tearing the bowel (one out of a thousand cases) or of excessive bleeding (three out of a thousand cases). It is also the most expensive of all the tests, so you need to check with your insurance company to see if it covers the procedure. (This is a good thing to do for any medical test.)

A virtual colonoscopy is a test that uses computer and radiology technology to simulate images of the complete colon on a screen without the use of an endoscope. (*Endoscopy* is the generic term for any procedure involving insertion of an instrument into an organ to view its interior, e.g., colonoscopy or sigmoidoscopy.) The accuracy of virtual colonoscopies has been good for larger polyps, but about 25 percent of polyps smaller than five millimeters in diameter may be missed. The test can only be used for diagnosis, and is especially useful if a colonoscopy is not possible. It requires the same bowel preparation as a regular colonoscopy. The gas pumped into the colon for the procedure can cause discomfort.

Recently, our ACE colorectal cancer survivors group asked a colorectal surgeon, Sharon Dykes, M.D., Ph.D., the following question: What do doctors really think about virtual colonoscopies? Dr. Dykes replied, "The virtual colonoscopy is likely the wave of the future as a screening tool for colorectal cancer and polyps, especially as graphics and imaging techniques become more definitive and powerful. Although promising, virtual colonoscopy is still a diagnostic test only. If polyps or other suspicious lesions are found, colonoscopy will be necessary for biopsy, removal, etc. In addition, issues have not been worked out regarding the timing of a colonoscopy after a positive virtual colonoscopy and also regarding personnel (endoscopy nurses, endoscopists, and endoscopy centers)."

Virtual colonoscopy could offer benefits as a new technology. It could reduce the number of colonoscopies used for diagnostic purposes and increase the number of colonoscopies performed therapeutically to remove polyps. Because virtual colonoscopy is new, it will likely be subject to continual improvement. Clearly, this is a subject colorectal cancer patients will want to continue exploring.

Missed Signals

While all of the above tests have merit, they are only effective if you pay attention to the results and to what you know about yourself. All positive tests should be followed up by a colonoscopy. If you continue to have symptoms or feel you have not had adequate testing, *you* must be the one to pursue further investigation, even if that means calling your physician again or going to another doctor.

At age forty-eight, Ruth, a production director in marketing, had to learn that lesson the hard way.

Ruth's Story

Ruth began having digestive problems—bloating, a change in bowel habits, and pain after eating. She underwent a sigmoidoscopy and a barium enema, neither of which indicated any problems. Physicians use both to screen for colon cancer, but at that time, nothing showed up. Her doctors believed she had irritable bowel syndrome.

Two years later, she began to have rectal bleeding, along with other symptoms. This time she was scheduled for a colonoscopy. Although no one really said "cancer" until after the tumor was removed and biopsied, that's when she got the news that changed her life. She found out she had colorectal cancer and that it had spread to her liver.

Her first reaction was fear. Then she asked, "Why me?" She continues, "I had been recently remarried, had a new grandchild, and worked at a job I loved as a production manager at an advertising agency. I felt that I didn't deserve to have this sort of upheaval cluttering my wonderful life. After shedding some tears, I made the conscious decision to wear my 'game face' for this experience. I knew that with almost every cancer, there were those people who survived, who beat it. Why shouldn't I be one of them?"

Four years later, Ruth is still cancer-free. Even with the missed signals, her cancer was arrested in time.

Risk Factors for Colorectal Cancer

When you are diagnosed with colorectal cancer, it's not unusual to feel some degree of fear, confusion, anger, and worry. This may be your first contact with your own mortality, and you might ask yourself, "How did I get here in the first place? Was there something about me that 'gave' me cancer?"

Research is ongoing and is always changing experts' ideas about what causes colorectal cancer. That said, certain risk factors increase a person's likelihood of getting the disease. These include the following:

- aging (90 percent of individuals diagnosed with colorectal cancer are over the age of fifty)

- family history (see "The Role of Genetics," on page 19)

- a personal history of colorectal cancer or polyps

- a diet high in fat and low in fruits and vegetables

- a sedentary lifestyle

- smoking

- heavy use of alcohol

- diabetes (diabetics are 30 to 40 percent more likely to develop colorectal cancer)

Some of these risk factors can be controlled. Changes in diet and lifestyle can lower the risks of developing colorectal cancer. The American Cancer Society recommends eating at least five servings of fruits and vegetables every day and several additional servings of foods from plant sources, limiting alcohol intake, giving up smoking, and exercising at least thirty minutes a day at least five days of the week. Dr. Rosy Daniel's suggestions in the chapter "Cleaning Up Your Act" in *The Cancer Prevention Book* are also wise and easy to follow (see Resources).

It must be emphasized, however, that the best protection against colorectal cancer comes from adequate screening. Almost all colorectal cancers develop from *adenomatous* (premalignant) polyps, so detecting these and having them removed can prevent cancer or prevent the cancer from spreading.

The Role of Stress

You may find you have well-meaning friends who actually become upset with you for "bringing this upon yourself." The implication is that you perhaps could have avoided cancer if you'd handled stress better. Be careful here. If you buy into this theory—and it is just a theory—then you may feel guilt in addition to all the other negative emotions that naturally arise at this time. There is no evidence of a cause-and-effect relationship between stress and colorectal cancer. What *has* been proven is that stress lowers the resistance of people fighting off any disease. Coping with stress in a positive way is one of the most helpful skills you can develop in order to bolster your immune system once you are diagnosed with colorectal cancer. Doing so will also help you deal more easily with the emotional ups and downs of the situation.

While there are plenty of books on the subject (a few of which are listed in the Resources at the back of this book), there is no single response to the challenge of handling stress. It is strongly recommended that you find some good methods for reducing stress and incorporate them into your life. Coping with stress at each stage of colorectal cancer is such a broad topic that a part of each chapter in this book addresses it, and all of Chapter 4 is devoted to the topic of dealing with your feelings. To start, here's a very simple yet highly effective technique for basic stress management.

Deep-Breathing Exercise

Experts consider paying attention to and consciously regulating your breathing a very effective way to reduce levels of stress and anxiety. Deep, slow breathing triggers the body's relaxation response, which is the opposite of the "fight-or-flight" response. Try to practice the following deep-breathing exercise every day. Before long, it will be like second nature to you to remember to slow down your breathing whenever you're feeling stressed and anxious about your health, or when you're undergoing a test that involves some physical discomfort.

- ◆ Ideally, set aside ten to thirty minutes for the exercise. However, you should still make time to practice even if you have only two or three minutes to spare. Find a quiet room and hang a "do not disturb" sign on the door. Sit or lie down comfortably.

- ◆ Close your eyes and repeat to yourself a comforting word or phrase, such as "relaxed," "peaceful," "nice and easy," "serene," "easy does it."

- ◆ Gradually slow down your breathing. Try the following pattern: Inhale for a count of four; then hold your breath for a count of four; next, exhale for a count of four; then hold without breathing for a count of four. Repeat several times.

- ◆ Make sure to breathe deeply, into your belly. Place one hand on your abdomen and the other on your chest. Your abdomen should expand while you inhale; your chest should barely move. As you exhale, let your abdomen flatten.

- ◆ If worries and distractions arise, don't hang on to them, but don't try to force them out of your mind, either. Simply allow them to float by, as if you were sitting on a riverbank watching your thoughts pass before you and keep going on downstream, out of your field of vision.

The Role of Genetics

As this book was being written, the media was paying much attention to the role genetics play in causing colorectal cancer. Our ACE support group from North Memorial Hospital asked Anna

Leininger, M.S., genetic counselor from the Minnesota Colorectal Cancer Initiative, to respond to the following questions:

Q. *How do genetics figure into colorectal cancer when 80 percent of colorectal cancer is not hereditary?*

A. All cancer is genetic, but not all cancer is hereditary. That might seem like a contradiction at first! Cancer is caused by damage to genes that control normal cell behavior. Normal cells follow rules of "cell etiquette." They reproduce responsibly and accurately, respect the "personal space" of neighboring cells, share available resources, stay where they belong, communicate with neighboring cells, and die when they wear out or become damaged. Genes control all of these behaviors. Cancer is caused by an accumulation of damage to these genes. When enough damage occurs, the cells grow without limit, take more than their fair share of available resources, invade surrounding tissues, and spread to other parts of the body. Colorectal cancer occurs when a series of four to seven "cell etiquette" genes become damaged over time. The genetic damage that causes most colorectal cancer occurs by chance or from environmental influences, accumulating over a lifetime.

People with a hereditary predisposition to developing colorectal cancer inherit a small degree of genetic damage at conception via the egg or sperm from the parents. The genetic instructions for one of the "cell etiquette" genes may be absent or faulty. Since the damage is present from conception, and all cells arise from that first cell, every cell in the body is one step closer to cancer. These people

- – may develop multiple colorectal polyps;
- – tend to develop polyps or cancer at earlier ages;
- – may have had colorectal cancer more than once, or have had another type of cancer;
- – may have a family history of colorectal polyps, colorectal cancer, or other types of cancer.

Q: *If there are other cancers in the family, should people wait until age fifty before being screened for colorectal cancer?*

A: It is not safe to wait until age fifty to begin colorectal screening if

- you have a close relative (parent, brother, sister, or child) who had a precancerous polyp or colorectal cancer before age sixty; or

- you have two close relatives who had precancerous colorectal polyps or colorectal cancer at any age.

In either of these cases, colorectal screening should begin at age forty or ten years prior to the earliest diagnosis of precancerous polyps (adenomas) or colorectal cancer in the immediate family, whichever is sooner. Colonoscopy should be the screening method. A family history of other types of cancer, such as lung, prostate, or breast cancer, usually does not affect your colorectal cancer risk.

A genetic evaluation should be scheduled to determine your risk and recommendations on an individual basis and to determine whether you are at risk for hereditary colorectal cancer if

- you or a family member had colorectal or endometrial cancer prior to age fifty;

- you or a family member had multiple colorectal polyps or other polyps before age forty;

- you or a family member had colorectal cancer more than once, or had colorectal cancer and another type of cancer; or

- you and/or several closely related family members have had colorectal polyps, colorectal cancer, or other types of cancer.

Screening should start earlier, should be repeated more frequently, and should be more thorough (colonoscopy) when cancer runs in the family. Screening for other types of cancer may be important in some families.

A genetic evaluation should be done by a physician, genetic counselor, or other medical professional with special training in genetics. You can find a genetic counselor by going to the following website: www.nsgc.org/resourcelink.asp.

Q: *Why do some seemingly healthy people who have always taken good care of themselves get cancer, while their siblings who drink, smoke, eat terribly, never take vitamins, etc., never develop any kind of cancer?*

A: Actually, there are at least two possible reasons for this. One reason is that cancer is caused by an accumulation of genetic damage, and genetic damage sometimes occurs by chance. By "doing all the right things," you can reduce but not eliminate the chances of genetic damage occurring. Another reason is that siblings do not share the exact same genetic content. On average, people have about half of their genes in common with each sibling. You may have different genes in common with different siblings. One sibling, for example, may have by chance inherited "versions" of genes that are more efficient at repairing DNA damage or breaking down toxic substances.

In theory, the actual amount of genetic material you have in common with each sibling may range from *no* genes in common to *all* genes in common. Statistically speaking, it is very unlikely that you would have *all* or *none* in common (like a coin coming up heads forty-six times in a row—once for each chromosome you inherited from each of your parents). But you may share fewer genes with some siblings than others. Only identical twins share all the same genes.

Q: *Can vitamins, herbs, etc., contribute to the prevention of colorectal cancer if there is a genetic predisposition to cancer?*

A: Little is known about how environmental factors or dietary supplements affect people with inherited colorectal cancer predisposition. It is not yet clear, for example, whether a low-fat, high-fiber, calcium-rich diet or exercise may help to prevent colorectal cancer in some people more than others, or whether people with a hereditary cancer predisposition are among those who may benefit from these kinds of measures. The National Cancer Institute is addressing questions such as this by funding the Early Detection Research Network High-Risk Registry. If you have an inherited cancer predisposition and would like to take part in this registry, you can contact researchers at Creighton University by calling (800) 648-8133, ext. 3189. Or go to http://medicine2.creighton .edu/EDRN-Registry.

Future discoveries about the links between genetics and colorectal cancer may impact prevention, diagnosis, and treatment, depending on the strengths and weaknesses found in an individual's genes. From studying gene alteration, oncologists (doctors specializing in the medical treatment of cancer) may be able to refine the selection of what type of chemotherapy works best in each individual case. Trials are underway that study how inserting genes into tumors may make them more responsive to certain medications.

❦ ❦ ❦

At the end of each chapter I've included a list of important points to take away from the chapter. Think of them as helpful things to do. Refer to the lists as needed once you've finished reading the book. You might even consider photocopying them and keeping them in a notebook for handy reference when you're planning doctor visits and scheduling tests. (See Chapter 3 for suggestions about keeping records and taking notes while you're planning and undergoing treatment.)

Here's the list for this chapter:

Positive Options for Facing the Unknown

◆ Listen to your instincts and don't let any embarrassment you might feel prevent you from going for a checkup.

- Pay attention to any unexplained bleeding or a change in bowel habits.

- Other warning signals, like bloating or minor fatigue, may be vague and hard to notice. All of these symptoms might be indicative of some other problem, but they need to be checked out immediately because of the possibility they are linked to cancer.

- To learn more about guidelines for screening, contact the Cancer Research and Prevention Foundation at (800) 227-2732 or visit its website at www.preventcancer.org/colorectal.

- Learn all you can about the tests you will be taking and any side effects you might experience from taking the tests. This may help make the situation less stressful. Be aware that you have a right to refuse to take any test.

- Talk to your doctor or your health-care provider if you feel you need more extensive testing. You may have to pay more money to undergo an additional test or to see another doctor, but doing so might be the right decision for you.

- Don't be afraid to talk to your doctor if you feel you need pain medication for a test.

- Use deep breathing as a way to relax if you become uncomfortable during a test. Sometimes counting can also help as a distraction. Practice the deep-breathing technique described in this chapter every day, and use it whenever you're feeling stressed or anxious about your health.

- Remember, despite the slight discomfort you may have to endure during tests, it's worth it to discover and arrest cancer at an early stage.

Chapter 2

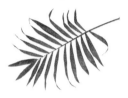

Gathering Information

If you have been diagnosed with colorectal cancer, you will be asked to undergo several more tests and procedures. The findings will help your doctors put together a treatment plan specifically for you. The emotional impact of going through tests and waiting for their results can be exhausting. Brenda Elsagher, comedienne and author of the book *If the Battle Is Over, Why Am I Still in Uniform?* endured moments of devastation and exasperation when she was diagnosed with colorectal cancer at age thirty-nine. Here is her story, as told in her book.

Brenda's Story

In the early days after receiving her diagnosis, Brenda tried to keep her sanity by rushing from each test back to work, pretending life was normal. Sometimes it helped to keep busy, and sometimes keeping busy only added to her stress.

As she remembers it, "Testing became a priority, and everything else revolved around that schedule. Hurry to this test, and then wait for the results. I was probed and scanned in parts of my body I never thought of as photogenic. Taking off from work during this testing time never entered my mind. I'm not sure if it was because of my mentality as a business owner and hairstylist. Money wasn't an issue, but I was concerned my clients might go to a new salon if testing took too much time from work. Fitting cancer into my calendar made me angry. I couldn't predict what my work days or hours would be. Cancer was not course work we ever studied in beauty school."

When she asked her doctor if her cancer had been detected early enough, he replied, "That is what we are going to find out through all these tests. If necessary, surgery will test the lymph nodes as well." So, with determination, she braved all the tests that were ordered. Each new test gave her and her doctor vital information.

Still, there were lighter moments during some of her ordeals. Brenda used her gift for comedy to make her health-care providers laugh when she told them jokes like this one: A patient had a cute young nurse who readied him for the test. He was in a tunnel-like machine for the time it takes the machine's recorder to say over and over, "Breathe in," "Breathe out," and "Hold your breath." When the test was completed and the patient was rolled out of the machine, he opened his eyes to see a much older nurse attending him. He commented, "I knew I was in there awhile, but I didn't know it was that long!"

❡ ❡ ❡

Humor, patience, keeping yourself busy, and the support of friends and family can all provide some relief from this emotionally draining experience. Try to stay in the present, and avoid jumping to conclusions. You have many options for treatment, which will be chosen based on the information received from your test results. This is an investigative period more than anything else, and just like going through any trial, new evidence will change the focus of your treatment. Understanding the purpose of each test and being prepared for the procedures involved can lessen their mystery. Be sure to ask your doctor if you can expect any side effects from each test you undergo.

Additional Tests for Colorectal Cancer

If cancer has been detected in your body, you will most likely undergo three additional tests: the rectal ultrasound, the CT scan, and the CEA blood tests.

The rectal ultrasound determines the depth of penetration of the cancer and whether or not it has metastasized (spread to other places in the body). This is another test that involves a long, flexible tube being inserted into the rectum. Usually you will be asked to prepare in advance for the procedure by taking two enemas at hourly intervals while you are still at home.

The test is performed at a minimally invasive unit of a hospital (sometimes called "short stay" or "day surgery"). You will be asked to lie in a fetal position on an examining table while a doctor inserts a well-lubricated endoscope into your rectum. High-frequency sound waves produce images that are projected onto a television-like screen.

The whole procedure is tolerable, but may produce some cramping. You may be helped by using deep breathing to relax (try the deep-breathing technique described in Chapter 1). You will be able to see the pictures of the ultrasound at the same time as the specialist; hopefully, you and your doctor will see no unwanted invaders.

The CT (computerized tomography) scan is actually composed of many X rays taken at various angles. It can produce images of organs that are difficult to see on regular X rays. You may be asked to fast before the test or to drink an iodine-based contrast agent. It is important that you tell your doctor beforehand if you are allergic to iodine.

The test is performed on an outpatient basis. You will be asked to move into many different positions while lying down, and you will be moved through an O-shaped X-ray machine. There is not much more to this test, other than following directions for holding your breath at intervals and remaining still.

The CEA (carcinoembryonic antigen) blood tests can indicate the presence of certain types of colorectal cancer, particularly if the cancer has spread to the liver. They are recommended for cancer patients to provide baseline information for your oncologist. While marker levels in a single CEA blood test could be elevated for reasons other than cancer, subsequent elevated levels send up a red flag calling for further investigation.

Stages of Colorectal Cancer

A diagnosis of cancer at any stage is disheartening. To determine the seriousness of the disease and to know the best way to treat it, medical experts use a system of "stages" to describe the progress of the cancer. A colorectal cancer is staged according to the characteristics of the tumor(s), how much the cancer has invaded the bowel, any involvement of the lymph nodes, and metastases to other organs. Interestingly, the size of a tumor is not as crucial to the patient's survival as its behavior.

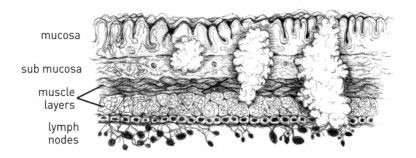

mucosa

sub mucosa

muscle layers

lymph nodes

Figure 2. Staging is determined by the degree of penetration of the tumor(s) into the bowel wall and whether the cancer has spread to the lymph nodes or other sites.

Your doctor will use one of three common staging systems, referred to as Duke's, MAC, and TNM. Ask your doctor to explain which system he or she is using and what each stage means in relation to your cancer. In general, regardless of which system is being used, the higher the number, the more dangerous the cancer. Here is a basic description of TNM, the most common staging system used by doctors, in which "T" stands for the primary tumor, "N" stands for lymph node metastasis, and "M" stands for distant metastasis.

Stage I: The cancer has not gone beyond the inner lining of the bowel. Monitoring and removal of polyps is usually all that is needed for care. Survival rates at this stage are in the 90 percent range.

Stage II: The cancer has gone beyond the wall of the colon and traveled to nearby tissue. In this case, surgical resection (removal of a portion) of the bowel is necessary; radiation and chemotherapy may be recommended.

Stage III: This is a more advanced stage wherein the cancer has invaded the lymph nodes. Resection, radiation, and/or *adjuvant* chemotherapy are necessary. (Adjuvant chemotherapy is chemotherapy that is used to augment or assist other procedures, such as surgery.) Survival rates at this stage are 30–70 percent for the first five years, if there is no recurrence.

Stage IV: Cancer is considered to be a stage IV if it has spread to or recurred in a distant site, such as the liver or the lung, a phenomenon called a *metastasis*. It is also considered a stage IV if it has recurred close to an original site, termed a *local recurrence*. The purpose of surgery at this stage is largely to relieve symptoms and prolong life, although some cancers can still be cured if only a few metastases are present and if surgery successfully removes all malignancy.

As testing progresses you may find that the stage you are diagnosed with will change. For instance, a colonoscopy may reveal a malignant polyp, which can be removed on the spot. If further tests indicate that the cancer cells have not raided other tissues, then you need no further treatment other than vigilant testing.

Adjusting to New Test Results

If you happen to find yourself diagnosed with cancer that is at an advanced stage, you need to keep in mind that statistics of survival are based on large groups of people. Interesting as they are, they do not represent you, as an individual. As a patient, with fear in my heart, I once asked Dr. Nemer, my colorectal surgeon, "What are my chances?" He replied, "One to 100 percent, because we are talking about you, and not a statistic." Remember, when you encounter dire statistics, that they are based on probabilities and may not apply to you at all.

Dan's Story

Dan could tell you that it's possible to beat the odds. One month after his twenty-fifth birthday, he found out he had stage IV colorectal cancer. He was dangerously anemic when he went into the emergency room. The first test they performed was a digital rectal exam and a stool sample (a fecal occult blood test).

He had never been in the hospital for anything, and in his words, "It scared the hell out of me. They did a bunch of blood work, and next they did a 'down the throat' scope looking for ulcers. Still, they had no answers. Finally, they gave me a colonoscopy."

At some point during the procedure the doctor asked Dan to look up at the screen. Reluctantly, he did. He describes what he saw as something "similar to the fat you cut off of chicken breasts. There was a lot of 'fat' everywhere. After a biopsy, I learned that it was pronounced cancer. This would explain the stomach flu I thought I had the last few weeks. Death filled my mind. At that moment, I accepted the possibility that I could die. After surgery, I found out the cancer had spread to my liver and twenty-some lymph nodes and that I had a 20 percent chance of making it to my thirtieth birthday."

Dan formed a mental picture of five people in his situation lining up on the "stage of life." Grimly, he realized that "Over the next five years, four of them would slowly exit, one at a time, with one left standing. Was that going to be me?"

Seven years later, Dan is still cancer-free. He feels that having a positive attitude was 90 percent of the battle. Now it is his turn to help others win, so he joined ACE and campaigns for others to undergo testing as soon as symptoms appear, even if they are still young. As he tells people, "Awareness is the key to beating this horrible disease. Listen to your body closely. You'd be surprised at what it is trying to tell you."

❡ ❡ ❡

While Dan's story is inspiring, there needs to be a word of caution here. It's common to experience negative feelings and fears at any stage of cancer. It's not possible to have a positive attitude all the time, and thinking positively is no guarantee of survival. However, developing your coping skills and embracing the best outlook you can will help you in your struggle. This is the time when finding a good support group or a counselor can ease the adjustment. Your doctor or a hospital social worker can refer you to appropriate resources for obtaining emotional and psychological support.

Questions from Colorectal Cancer Patients

As colorectal cancer survivors, we know that information about our disease empowers us to make better decisions. Our ACE support group posed the following questions to colorectal surgeons Amy Thorsen, M.D., and Karim Alavi, M.D., from Colon and Rectal Associates Ltd.

Q: *Why do some colorectal cancers develop with symptoms and others do not?*

A: (*Dr. Thorsen*) Most colorectal cancers are asymptomatic. Symptoms may become more apparent in larger tumors and in tumors closer to the rectum. Colon cancers can bleed; if the tumor is in the right side of the colon (far from the rectum), it may only manifest as anemia or microscopic blood in the stool. Cancers of the rectum and the left side of the colon may lead to symptoms of bright-red rectal bleeding because the blood travels through less colon and does not get reabsorbed.

As colon cancers get larger, they can cause blockages in the colon. Since the left colon is smaller in diameter and the stool is more formed at this point, obstruction is more likely to occur in left-sided cancers. Some obstructing tumors will let only liquid stool get by, whereas others cause a narrowing of the stool.

Q: *Why do doctors still perform flexible sigmoidoscopy? With so much colon cancer now being found further up in the colon, the procedure seems like a waste of time and money.*

A: *(Dr. Alavi)* It is important to point out that flexible sigmoidoscopy still has a place in screening and surveillance. There are now two currently accepted methods for screening colon cancer: flexible sigmoidoscopy every five years, combined with an annual fecal occult blood test. This has proven to be effective for identifying the majority of colon cancers. More and more polyps are being found in the right side of the colon. If we believe in the polyp-to-cancer sequence, then colonoscopy would be more useful, as polyps could be removed during the test. That is why physicians are increasingly recommending a screening colonoscopy for their patients.

Q: *How can colorectal cancer move to other organs such as the lungs, breast, and brain and still be considered colorectal cancer?*

A: *(Dr. Alavi)* Colon cancer can metastasize (move to another part of the body) to other organs, particularly to the lungs, liver, adrenal glands, and sometimes the brain. The cancer starts out at the mucosa, or inner lining of the colon. Once it penetrates the first muscle layer, it becomes exposed to lymphatics (vessels carrying lymph fluid) and blood vessels, which then carry these cells to other organs. Once the cancer cells reach their destination, they grow and form tumor deposits, but since the cells originated in the colon, the cancer type is still considered colorectal.

Q: *Is there any concrete evidence to support the "environment" factor in cancer? Is there anything we should be doing to change our environment to prevent cancer?*

A: *(Dr. Alavi)* There are numerous factors that are involved in the development of colon cancer. These include, in no specific order, genetics, polyps, history of inflammatory bowel disease, diet (particularly diets high in unsaturated fats and low in calcium), and others. This list only demonstrates that there are numerous factors involved; to date, no single initiating event has been demonstrated. Recent studies have shown promise that diets rich in calcium and fiber help reduce the development of polyps and, thus, cancer. Additional studies have suggested that taking a small daily dose of aspirin can also reduce the incidence of colorectal cancer. Clearly, more work needs to be done in these areas.

❡ ❡ ❡

Colorectal surgeon Sharon Dykes, M.D., Ph.D., answered the following questions about colonoscopies and the accuracy of tumor markers given to colorectal cancer patients:

Q: *What should I say to a general practitioner or other primary-care physician who won't recommend a colonoscopy?*

A: If you are fifty years of age and currently have no symptoms associated with colon cancer (abdominal pain, bleeding, change in bowel habits, or weight loss), then it is appropriate to request a referral for colonoscopy for screening purposes. If you have any of the symptoms mentioned above, it is appropriate to request referral for a colonoscopy as symptoms arise. If your practitioner will not make a referral for colonoscopy, then schedule an office visit with a colorectal surgeon to discuss your concerns.

Q: *Are the tumor marker tests (like the CEA) that colorectal cancer patients take able to detect all types of tumors?*

A: Tumor markers, in general, are substances that may be produced by both cancerous and noncancerous tissues. Therefore, the presence of an elevated tumor marker level may suggest, but is not specific for, cancer development. In addition, most tumor markers are associated with specific types of cancers, and thus the tests will not detect all types of cancers.

Myths and Misinformation

When you are gathering information, you need to be aware of where the information comes from. Myths can be life threatening when they influence you to act in ways that are destructive to your health. If you are a woman and believe women are not susceptible to colorectal cancer, you may fail to ask for adequate screening as part of your routine health plan. If you think this disease only happens to older people, you may ignore symptoms that should be addressed. If you believe colorectal cancer is impossible to overcome, you may fail to take life-saving measures to counteract the progression of your illness. Discussed below are a few of the more common myths that can obstruct getting proper treatment, as well as some truths to counteract the myths:

Myth: *Colorectal cancer is a disease of men and the elderly.*

Truth: *Men and women are almost equally at risk. Colorectal cancer can occur at any age.*

The median age when colorectal cancer occurs is sixty-two, but people under age forty get colorectal cancers too. Both men and women are equally at risk. This year it is estimated that more than fifty-six thousand people in the United States will die from colorectal cancer, twenty-eight thousand of them women.

A classic study conducted by Stanford University of two hundred women ages forty-one to ninety-five in the San Francisco Bay Area revealed that women underestimated the risks of their getting colorectal cancer and overestimated the dangers of breast cancer. Women were more likely to go for routine mammograms and were uninformed about screening guidelines for colorectal cancer. The study concluded that many of these women did not get screened because they perceived colorectal cancer as a man's disease.

Myth: Colorectal cancer is usually fatal.

Truth: Most colorectal cancers can be cured if caught early enough.

This myth could prove harmful if patients believe there is no hope and that cancer will take their life no matter what they do. Such beliefs may cause them not to seek the help they need to overcome the disease.

Ninety percent of Stage I colon cancer patients will be considered "cured," meaning the patient is still alive without a recurrence, if after five years the cancer has not spread *at all* beyond its original site. Even if the cancer has metastasized (spread to a regional or distant site from where it originated), recovery rates can be impressive for cancers that are aggressively treated with surgery and nonsurgical treatments, such as radiation or chemotherapy.

Myth: If you don't have a history of colorectal cancer in your family, you don't have to be concerned about getting the disease.

Truth: This belief can be dangerous because it might lull people into thinking that they are immune from colorectal cancer, and they might fail to get proper screening.

No one knows exactly what causes colorectal cancer, but genetic factors predispose a person to be susceptible to the disease.

Since most colorectal cancers originate from polyps, people with a family history of inflammatory disease or of *hereditary non-polyposis colon cancer* (referred to as HNPCC) are at a much greater risk of developing colorectal cancer. Another condition called *familial adenomatous polyposis* (FAP) drastically increases the risk that some of the polyps will become cancerous. However, although heredity plays an important role in colorectal cancer, two-thirds of colorectal cancers occur in people with no significant history of the disease in their family.

Myth: *Don't get too close to a cancer patient; it's catching.*

Truth: *You may have a genetic predisposition toward getting colorectal cancer, but it is not spread by contact or by being close to someone who has the disease.*

Emotionally, this myth could be harmful to your relationships.

Cancer patients need reassurances, not people backing away from them.

Myth: *Doctors and the American Cancer Society are in a conspiracy against new advances in medicine because they want to hold on to their jobs.*

Truth: *This doesn't make much sense for various reasons. Doctors are overworked. Those who are salaried through health plans, group organizations, or government service are paid the same whether or not their patients are sick. Keeping their patients healthy would only lessen their workload, not enhance their income.*

This myth is particularly poisonous because it could destroy the patient-physician trust so necessary for good care and lead the patient to consult unreliable resources.

Many myths and much misinformation are spread through word of mouth and by some questionable media sources wanting a sensational news story to bolster their circulation. If you have questions about your disease, consult qualified medical personnel or another reliable resource, such as the American Cancer Society or the National Cancer Institute. The Internet is full of both good information and misinformation. Beware of easy cures and false promises.

Positive Options when Gathering Information

◆ Keep your mind open to new ideas and options as you gather information.

- Become as well informed as you can about your stage of cancer. Knowledge empowers you to make better decisions. The American Cancer Society and the National Cancer Institute publish pamphlets that are loaded with information. The Web can also be a good source of information to a discerning consumer. These sources can supplement the information you will receive from your doctors.

- Get some help to adjust to your new diagnosis. Consider obtaining psychological and emotional support by joining a cancer survivors' group or seeing a professional counselor.

- Remember that statistics are based on groups. You are an individual.

- Go to reliable sources for answers to your questions.

- Beware of myths and misinformation. They could influence you to act in ways that may be destructive to your health.

Chapter 3

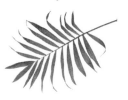

Working with Medical Professionals to Develop a Health Plan

During the Depression, my grandfather was the only doctor for the people of Sandstone, a small town in northern Minnesota. If patients couldn't pay in money, they would give him a chicken, a bag of wheat, or whatever they could. When the first hospital was built in town, it was dedicated to him. I grew up with a tremendous respect for the medical profession.

When I was coping with colorectal cancer, I had a medical team that gave me excellent care. My high regard for doctors continued. Most of the members of our ACE group also had good experiences with their physicians and medical teams. Nevertheless, for any patient dealing with medical professionals, problems or considerations can arise that you need to confront.

After a diagnosis of colorectal cancer, you will find yourself facing not only emotional decisions but also practical ones. These can include medical, financial, and legal concerns. Don't let the complexities overwhelm you. It might help to remember that you are a consumer and are buying health-care. You wouldn't dream of building a house without enlisting the help of a qualified contractor whom you trust. Communication with your medical team is a top priority. You need to find someone you can easily work with to develop a well-thought-out plan for your care. Other experts might need to be consulted, and you need to become your own best advocate. Get involved in your own care to develop a health plan suited to your needs.

Legal and Financial Concerns

The last thing you need, when diagnosed with colorectal cancer, is to have uncertainty about your job, your health insurance, or your finances. These matters need to be clarified at the beginning of your journey with cancer, so don't procrastinate in dealing with them.

If You Are Employed

Inform your employer or your human resources office of your diagnosis, and find out what options you have if it becomes necessary for you to take time off for future treatments or appointments. As an employee, you have certain rights that are protected by law. Being aware of them can help you plan your life. Some of these laws are briefly outlined below:

- The Consolidated Omnibus Budget Reconciliation Act of 1985 (COBRA) stipulates that if you lose your job or have your working hours reduced, you may be entitled to continuation of the medical insurance at your own cost at the group rates you had with your (former) employer for a period of eighteen months or longer, depending on the circumstances.

- Under the Americans with Disabilities Act (ADA), you have some employment safeguards and cannot be dismissed or demoted solely because you have cancer. It applies to companies with fifteen or more employees.

- The Family and Medical Leave Act (FMLA) allows you twelve weeks of annual leave to attend to your health care or to act as caretaker for someone in your family who is very sick. Note that it applies to companies with fifty or more employees.

Dealing with Medical Insurance

If you are covered by a health-insurance plan, you need to have a clear understanding of what steps you must take to have a procedure or treatment preapproved. Most plans will encourage you to get a second opinion shortly after you've been diagnosed and will be willing to cover your expenses for doing so. Getting a second opinion is your right as a patient and should not be a problem. The plan will usually require you to see a doctor who is part of its network.

If you have any questions, most plans have a patient representative you can call. Contact your medical insurance provider or your employer's human resources department to obtain the phone number for the patient representative, and write it down. This person can help you through a maze of misunderstandings.

If your employer offers an open-enrollment period, which typically means you will be able to change your coverage without the need for a physical examination or the completion of a questionnaire about your medical history, you may consider taking this option for a better plan at this time.

Read carefully through each piece of correspondence you get from your health-insurance company. You might receive a bill concerning a test or procedure that was deemed necessary by your doctor, or there may be some questions concerning treatment or the type of test you were asked to take.

You may be responsible for paying more of certain bills than you anticipated. This can be stressful in itself. (Here's another area where the stress-management techniques you've been learning can help you keep your cool.) There are some actions you can take right now, before problems occur. Contact your insurance carrier to find out what is covered and whether or not you need to be referred to a specialist by your primary doctor. When considering which specialists to see, "in network" or "preferred provider" are key words to look for if you're working with a managed-care plan.

If you have no insurance, you need to check with your local social services regarding the availability of any government-assistance programs. If you are eligible, call Medicare. Securing financial help if you are an uninsured patient is one of the unfortunate, unsolved puzzles that has to be worked out in today's world. If you are eligible for Medicare or Medicaid benefits, you may want to contact an appropriate local Social Security agency to find out if you should supplement your plan. If you become disabled before full retirement age with an impairment that will prevent you from doing substantial work for a year or more, and if you have earned enough work credits, you can apply for Social Security Disability Income. In either case, contact the Social Security Administration and ask to receive its free booklet on these topics. (See Resources for contact info.)

Managing Medical Records

As your care becomes more complex, it becomes very important to keep proper records. Doing so is important both so you can easily access the information for your own purposes and so you can readily submit the necessary forms to insurance companies. It's a good idea to request a copy of all medical records and bills from your health-care providers. Typically, you need the following information whenever you visit a new doctor for the first time:

- health-insurance policies and resources
- phone numbers for health insurance and/or Medicare, Medicaid
- phone numbers and addresses of doctors, clinics, and hospitals
- phone numbers and addresses of local pharmacies
- records of past significant medical history

- lists of all prescription medications that you are currently taking

- lists of all nonprescription medications, supplements, and herbal remedies you're currently taking (since some herbal preparations interact strongly with pharmaceuticals)

- lists of allergies

- a copy of your health-care directive, if applicable. Sometimes referred to as an "advanced directive" or living will," this document clarifies to family members and health-care providers what your wishes are should your illness progress in such a way that you become unable to communicate for yourself.

Store other health-related data at home. Keep all of your records in one place, such as a drawer or file cabinet, preferably one that's fireproof. Be sure to list specific dates and procedures, prescriptions and dosages, dates of phone calls, and a log of conversations. Note all of your appointments on a calendar, specifying time, doctor, and procedure.

Finding a Good Doctor

Part of a well-coordinated plan involves finding the right doctor to be the lead member of your team. You need to take an active part in this selection. A good doctor can act as a strategist, directing you to the right personnel and resources and helping you with the logistics.

Be selective when choosing your doctor. You have a right to choose someone who you feel is the best for your situation. This may mean that, after meeting with one doctor, you will want to go to another doctor or get a second opinion. It's important to select someone whom you feel comfortable with on a personal level. This can be extremely helpful in reducing some of your stress. As my ACE colleagues will attest, when we entered into the new category of "cancer patient," most of us were given top-level care. Most of the time we were lucky to be referred to professionals who suited us well. Some people were not so lucky, and years later are still lamenting that they didn't switch doctors at the very beginning.

Here's a short list of qualities you will want in all of your doctors. Think of these as the equivalent of a soldier's C rations—they will provide you with sustenance when you are in the trenches, so to speak:

- competence

- conscientiousness

- communication skills

- concern

- compatibility

Keep in mind that not all colorectal cancers involve extensive surgery. Don't panic if you are referred to a colorectal surgeon once you have been diagnosed with cancer. A colorectal surgeon is a doctor who is an expert in the surgical and nonsurgical treatment of colon and rectal problems. Being referred to one does not mean you are automatically going to need an operation. Even if a polyp is malignant, more surgery may be unnecessary after the polyp is removed. To locate a board-certified colorectal surgeon in your area, ask your present doctor or call the National Cancer Institute (NCI) at (800) 422-6237.

When a major consultation is scheduled with any doctor, it's a good idea to take someone you trust along to your appointment. Aside from that person being an added source of support, it's helpful to have another set of ears present. You need to have a clear understanding of what the doctor is saying, and it's hard to keep your emotions from interfering with your ability to listen. Take along a small notebook, and write down specific words that can be looked up in a dictionary later.

As cancer survivors, we have generally become more understanding about how hard it can be to get a doctor's appointment. We have learned that it's very sick people who are filling up those time slots. This is especially true of a doctor dealing with cancer patients. One thing to keep in mind: Always, always be as nice to the receptionists in your doctors' offices as you can be. First of all, they're probably overworked; secondly, they have power, and you want them on your side, especially when it comes to scheduling appointments with a busy doctor. It doesn't make any more sense to tell off a receptionist than it would to scold a traffic cop. With both, being unpleasant gives you diminishing returns.

How to Get the Best Results when Working with Doctors and Nurses

Jane Nielsen, a cancer patient and oncology nurse whom we met in Chapter 1, has seen both sides of the dilemmas people face when trying to work out health issues. She offers the following excellent advice for patients: "Advocate for what you need, but do so in a manner that honors your doctors' time. By taking the time to be organized and finding out how the offices of your respective doctors function, you increase the cooperation factor, and thus increase the probability that you will get the answers you request. Remember that you are part of the treatment team and part of the solution, not part of the problem."

Jane has written the following list of practical tips to get you started:

1. Purchase a standard three-ring binder and a three-hole punch. Fill the notebook with lined paper, index sheets or section dividers, and pocket folders. This is your communication center. Store in it everything you are given that has relevance to your care: diagnostic test instructions, lab results, after-care guidelines, receipts, notes from office visits, and your journal.

2. Journal your physical and emotional status in a brief, matter-of-fact form that is easy to review and share with your doctor or health-care team. (You may wish to record the details of your journey to recovery in a separate journal

you keep by your bedside.) Doctors need to know when a symptom or complication began and how long it has lasted. For example, was the pain constant, episodic, sharp, dull, aching, or burning? How would you rate the pain on a zero-to-ten scale, if zero is pain-free?

3. Write down questions for upcoming visits, leaving space for the answers you will receive. Condense and prioritize the questions, so that if the doctor is called away during your visit, you will have gotten the most important part of your agenda addressed.

4. Whenever possible, take a family member or friend with you to be another set of ears. They can take notes during your visits, so you can do something very critical: listen. Doctors prefer to clarify information during the visit, rather than receive calls after hours. Understandably, it is sometimes difficult to interrupt and ask what an unfamiliar term means. In such cases, use hand signals, such as "time-out," to prompt the doctor to pause. Then take the opportunity to say, "I didn't understand the word you just used, could you explain it?"

5. Develop a respectful, courteous relationship with nurses and office staff. Find out the names of the people you talk to. Ask for the phone numbers you may need to call during or after hours to report side effects of medication or complications of treatment. There are usually specific staff members who make appointments and/or preauthorize patients for special tests and therapy. Find out their names. Ask about their policy for filling cancellations, about the notification procedure, and if there is a waiting list. Ask before you need to know, so that in a time of stress you can save yourself and the staff valuable time.

6. Before phoning your doctor's office to ask for anything, write down exactly what you plan to say, beginning with your name and phone number, and a brief description of

what you need. This script is critical to getting the results you need. It honors your doctor's time and enables the phone personnel to process your information. When making your phone call, you may end up leaving your message on a machine with limited recording space. Speak slowly. Say your name, then spell it, provide your date of birth, and leave the number(s) where you can be reached. Summarize your request. Don't give details.

7. Avoid aggressive, emotionally charged communication with your medical team. You may be fighting cancer, but you don't want to alienate your caregivers in the process. Be honest, but be tactful and factual. Avoid power struggles. Clashes drain you of precious energy and sabotage cooperation. Remember, doctors and nurses are human. Just as you are not always at your best, they get worn down, also. Make tolerance, patience, and a sense of humor your best allies.

8. Determine whom you want to give access to your medical information, and sign appropriate releases. Privacy laws restrict health-care personnel from talking to anyone who is not listed on your consent form. Even if your spouse or adult children always accompany you to doctors' visits, without your *written* consent, they cannot legally be given information over the phone when they call on your behalf. Ask for copies of any consents for your file. Place one in your notebook, and give copies to the individuals participating in your care.

9. Finally, remember to say "thank you" and to express your appreciation for service rendered. Your health-care team is typically overworked and underappreciated. Let kindness be the mortar in the foundation of this critical, supportive relationship. Surprise them with thank-you notes, candy, fresh salsa and chips, or flowers from your garden. You will touch their heart, and they will never forget you!

Keep in mind that differences in personalities may be the cause of some clashes. Some people want a doctor to make all their decisions for them, and some doctors are perfectly willing to do just that. In extreme cases, this kind of doctor will discourage you from seeking information elsewhere or from asking too many questions. On the other hand, bringing too much information to doctors can be distracting and take too much time. If you have something you wish your doctor to read, it might be better to send it to the office before your visit along with a small note of explanation. A well-researched article from a reliable resource will have more validity. If you have a lengthy subject you need to talk to your doctor about, make an extra appointment for a consultation. Doctors generally have a short time period of time for seeing each patient, and you want to make every moment count.

Some highly qualified doctors may be aloof and give you the impression that whatever decisions you make are in your hands and not their concern. Dealing with that sort of attitude may be too great a burden for you at this point. You may feel totally inadequate when it comes to making any important decisions regarding your care. This is the time for you to contact a patient representative at the hospital.

If all else fails, even at this point, it might be better for you to begin seeing another doctor. This is a team you are putting together, and if there is too much dissonance for you and your physician to work together, now is the time to change.

Learning the Language of Medicine Land

In the months ahead, it is going to be imperative that you speak the same language as your care providers. The quickest way to find out what doctors, nurses, or technicians are saying is to simply *ask them*. Medical terminology can sound like a foreign language, and there may be times when you need to ask your healthcare provider to write down the words or help you pronounce them. This isn't a pointless exercise. It is important to be able to tell other caregivers what test, medication, or procedure you have been given.

Sometimes the words used can be confusing. When talking about blood, *occult* means "hidden" and does not refer to the supernatural. *Benign* means "good" and *malignant* means "bad," or cancerous. It might seem like doublespeak to call a bad test "positive" and a good test "negative," but that's the way it works.

What We Would Like to Say to Doctors

Here are some things our ACE group would like doctors to know:

"Remember, always, that you are working with a human being who has cancer."

"We know you are busy, but one-minute management can work wonders. Take a moment to explain to us that you are leaving town and how to get in touch with another doctor in case of an emergency. Let us know when you think we are doing a good job in combating our disease. Say hello."

"Don't bludgeon us with too many medical terms. We don't want to know how much you know, only to simply understand what you are saying."

"A clear explanation of a procedure or the scope of our disease will help to demystify what we are encountering. We want to be educated."

"Be honest with us, but bad news can be delivered kindly. We don't want to be placated by false hopes or devastated by bleak prophecies, when neither may prove to be true."

"Treat us as you would want to be treated, with respect and with regard for our dignity."

"Both or one of us may not always be at our best, and there may be times when we ruffle each other's feathers. If we practice good communication, we can put these times into perspective. A little humor and consideration will go a long way."

Positive Options for Working with Medical Professionals to Develop a Health Plan

◆ Find the best doctor you can who is well suited to your needs, and take an active role on your medical team. If you have medical insurance, be sure the doctor you choose is part of your network of preferred providers.

◆ You have a right to a second opinion if you want one. Call your insurance company and talk to the patient representative about how to arrange for a second opinion or ask your doctor for a referral.

◆ Take along another person when consulting the doctor, and ask her or him to take notes. You can look up unfamiliar words later.

◆ Ask your doctor or your nurses to explain any terminology you don't understand.

◆ Contact your insurance company and your employer to inform them of your circumstances. Find out what options you are entitled to if you need time off for tests and medical appointments.

◆ Keep all of your records in one place, like a drawer or a file. Note all of your appointments on a calendar, according to time, doctor, and procedure.

◆ Develop a courteous, cooperative working arrangement with your health professionals. Be respectful of their time.

◆ My *Medical Journal* (by Judy McElwain, R.N., and Gail Bernier) is an excellent guide for helping you organize your personal medical information. For ordering information, e-mail Info@Health-Text.com.

Chapter 4

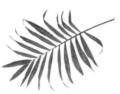

Dealing with Your Feelings

No one gets through life without experiencing some grief. Although people usually think of grief as connected with end-of-life issues, significant bereavement also occurs when someone is going through cancer. Indeed, feelings of loss affect not only patients but also the people who care about them.

Coping with a Diagnosis of Cancer

When diagnosed with cancer, people generally feel some combination or progression of anger, denial, depression, bargaining, and acceptance, all of which are basic and necessary stages of the grieving process. Colorectal cancer, by its very nature, can be hard to talk about, especially when it comes to your feelings and day-to-day struggles. As mentioned earlier, you may want to consider joining a support group or talking to a counselor (see page 56 for things to think about when looking for a support group).

You may be upset about health setbacks, usually brought about through side effects of cancer treatments. Though these are often temporary, you may feel that you have lost your good health forever. You may be worried about the emotional losses that could come from friends or loved ones temporarily distancing themselves from you. You may fear that your life will never be the same again.

To begin with, keep in mind this old adage: Never say never. When I felt my worst, an old friend told me, "This too shall pass." I want to pass that message along to you—it was helpful to me, and I gradually began to have better days both in my health and outlook. Remember, too, that good things can come out of negative situations.

You are about to learn new dimensions of the word coping. If you have successfully handled difficulties earlier in your life, the skills you learned and used then will come to your aid now. You will be challenged like you never have been before. You will find that you are learning new ways to deal with almost any problem you may encounter in the future. That's not bad.

Cancer seems to attract a network of caring individuals. Be prepared to discover that some of the most seemingly indifferent people will surprise you. Be ready to accept random acts of kindness from people you hardly know. On the other hand, people you love the most may find it hard to be close to you at this time. Keep in mind that they are afraid too.

Anger as a Catalyst

Anger is not an uncommon response to learning that you have colorectal cancer. After all, your life is being disrupted, your plans may need to be put on hold, and you have lost the confidence you once had in your healthy immune system. That's quite a load.

Stifling your anger takes up the energy you need to survive. It may be wiser for you to vent your feelings to a caring listener in a situation designed for that purpose. Attend a support group, schedule an appointment with an individual counselor, or express yourself to a trusted friend or family member. If you decide to lean on someone close to you for emotional support, make sure the "ground rules" are set up so that you also respect the needs of the listener.

You may be able use anger to your advantage. Let it fuel your resolve to be proactive about setting up the best health-care plan for your specific needs. Let it spur you to get help right away for dealing with your emotions. The key objective here, however, is to reduce the anger rather than feed it. Otherwise, chronic, unresolved anger will eventually take its toll and work against your healing.

Denial as a Form of Protection

Denial may help you temporarily cope with a situation until you are more ready to face it head-on. When I was first diagnosed with stage III cancer, I remember looking at the images being transmitted during a rectal ultrasound. My attention was fixed on three dark spots I surmised were the malignant tumors. The room became very quiet. The lighthearted kidding ended. The only sound was the beeping of the machine, which I felt was announcing bad news. Dr. Finne's silence told me he was reluctant to announce the results. When he started to plot quadrants over the three dreaded, dark invaders, I succumbed to despair. My body stiffened. In a sympathetic, soft voice, he said, "It looks like your cancer has invaded some of your lymph nodes." He explained that he would have to cut off a little of each node to have it biopsied. "This isn't going to be easy. Hang on," he apologized.

His snipping didn't hurt, really. Maybe I was just numb, but I didn't feel any physical pain as he went through the business of removing pieces from my rectum. I lay there, in complete denial, as we discussed my future.

"As I told you before," he said, "if the tests come out positive, you're going to need a resection, radiation, and chemotherapy."

I tried to respond, to organize my thoughts during those moments by groping for the familiar routines I desperately wanted to use to protect me. I explained how I couldn't take time off at this point because I was really needed at school, plus I was busy planning for my daughter Laura's wedding in five months.

Dr. Finne wasn't buying any of it. Quietly, he said, "You need to take care of your health first, you know."

I knew that what he was saying made sense. I knew that my life had taken a solemn turn. I knew that to deny the danger would be the worst thing I could do.

It seems trivial now, but the first question I asked was, "Will I lose my hair?" The thought of losing my hair was excruciating. I couldn't think beyond that to ask any other questions about more serious issues.

"Probably not," he responded. "Not with the chemo you take for this kind of cancer, but an oncologist will be able to tell you more."

An oncologist. I was going to have to see an oncologist. The words *chemo, radiation,* and *resection* were echoing in my mind like part of a bad dream.

I found myself still fighting facts. I left, desperately hoping, in spite of what we'd seen on the screen, that the black dots would turn out benign. After all, I'd had close calls before with questionable mammograms.

I spent the next two days in denial, waiting for the final results. I sensed I was in deep trouble, but I wasn't going to accept that fact until I actually knew for sure. This state of mind has some positive value, because waiting in limbo for the results of a test can be excruciating. In some ways, waiting is worse than the actual ordeal. Almost more than anything else, I wanted the waiting to be over.

At 9:00 A.M., as I stood in front of my class, the phone rang. I told the students to begin to fill out their worksheets as I answered the call. It was Dr. Finne. He asked, "Is this a good time to talk?" I should have replied, "No," but I was too anxious to wait any longer.

"I'm sorry to tell you this," he said, "but we got the results back on your ultrasound, and the cancer has metastasized to some of the adjacent lymph nodes, so we're going to have to begin a program of radiation and chemotherapy immediately and then schedule you for a resection."

The cancer had spread to my lymph nodes. He would call Dr. Nemer, my colorectal surgeon, immediately. I weakly replied that I understood what he was saying. He ended the conversation by telling me with conviction, "I want you to know we're going to fight this."

I hung up the phone and faced the truth. The good health I had taken for granted had broken down. I had to undergo major repairs in order to survive.

I didn't know enough at that point to even ask the right questions. Getting informed would be my first line of attack, I reasoned, so I spent the next few days reading all I could on colorectal cancer.

That was how I confronted the situation. However, my husband Dave's way of dealing with the anxiety was quite the opposite. He was struggling with all of the recent happenings and had been significantly deprived of sleep for a few days. While I obsessively searched for information, he desperately needed to get some rest, so he took long naps. When we finally started to talk about how we were going to spend the next few months, he told me he wasn't convinced that I had heard the doctor correctly and that it just couldn't be as bad as I imagined. Didn't I, after all, go in to see the doctor almost immediately when I first started to spot? Didn't the doctor tell us on our first consultation that I would be put on only a watchful schedule of tests? Maybe the colorectal surgeon wouldn't agree with what the other doctor was saying. Maybe the ultrasound wasn't all that accurate.

This conversation was maddening to me. I wanted to believe my husband's version of the situation, but I needed to face reality. I was preparing for my battles, and he was telling me there wasn't a war. When I said that I could probably keep teaching until spring vacation but might need to take a medical leave until next year, he thought I was jumping the gun and misinterpreting the facts. He wanted to wait and hear what the colorectal surgeon had to say.

Thank goodness for the all the counselors in my life who have taught me to take care of myself in situations like this. Through some flash of insight, I realized that we were both afraid, only we were reacting to the news in different ways. In times of extreme stress, considerable strain is put on a relationship because of the conflicting ways that people need to deal with their fears. You will likely find it particularly hard to talk about your cancer diagnosis with the people you love. Don't think of it as a one-time conversation. It needs to be ongoing and timely. It's important that your children, even your adult children, hear the latest news from you rather than from someone else. As much as possible, involve your children in your care. Perhaps allow them to make a special meal for you or give you a massage. At the time of your diagnosis, family members need to feel loved and be given assurances, just as much as you do.

Bargaining for Time

Most of us are unprepared for a diagnosis of colorectal cancer. One of the reactions people have is to bargain with doctors to buy more time before having surgery or beginning treatments. Other concerns immediately take over when you are first told what procedures you might need to undergo. You might remember personal obligations or plans to do something else. Taking time off for your health was not on your calendar.

Julie's Story

When Julie experienced sporadic changes in her bowel habits, she ignored the signals for almost eight years. It was easy to write off the symptoms to stress, hemorrhoids, or perhaps to a condition called irritable bowel syndrome. She was busy trying to establish herself as an actress while also working in the claims department at a national insurance company. Eventually, the pain caught up with her. Blood and mucus in her stools plus unusual, tubular bowel movements convinced her she had to have a more thorough examination. She contacted a colorectal surgeon and shortly thereafter was given a flexible sigmoidoscopy. The results floored her.

With a sense of urgency, her doctor told her, "I'd stake my reputation on the fact that this is cancer, and I'm sure the pathology report will support my diagnosis." He advised her not to wait any longer than two weeks to have surgery. Julie protested. She was enjoying a successful run in a starring role in the comedy *How to Talk Minnesotan*, and her understudy was going on vacation.

"I really can't take the time off until she comes back," she explained.

Her doctor looked her square in the eye and said in no uncertain terms, "This is cancer. The pathology report will confirm this, but I know what I'm looking at. I do over a hundred of these sigmoidoscopies a year. We have to get this out within two weeks."

Julie tried to protest that she needed more time.

"Two weeks," the doctor persisted. "You can only wait two weeks."

Julie is a warrior, and she bravely confronted her diagnosis head-on, but when she told her understudy about the dilemma she was in, she burst into tears. Still, something told her she would overcome cancer and be a "thriver," not just a survivor. Although she wanted to delay the surgery, she quickly went ahead with it because she also knew that she wanted to enjoy a long life.

She knows now how lucky she was to get into surgery when she did. A tumor the size of a key lime was found and removed, along with twenty-two lymph nodes. Although she endured some significantly adverse side effects while taking chemotherapy, the cancer was encapsulated, so she remains a stage II colorectal cancer patient with no recurrences four years later.

Today, besides continuing her career in acting and working for the insurance company, Julie organizes a cadre of speakers for ACE and frequently gives talks to businesses and conferences. She effectively conveys the difficulty of being a patient and of facing a cancer diagnosis. She feels lucky to have had exceptionally caring people help her through the experience. At the end of each talk, Julie has a strong message to deliver to doctors and others in the medical profession: "Please never forget that you are treating a human being with cancer. Kindness and a regard for the dignity of the patient should never be forgotten."

Sorrow vs. Depression

No matter how brave a front people put up when confronting cancer, you can be reasonably sure it will hit them hard emotionally. Ruth Edstrom's expression of putting on her "game face" describes many of us who are trying to control the grief we feel inside. I look back now at a page from a journal I wrote while gazing out over Lake Superior just after my diagnosis changed from stage I to stage III. It will give you an idea of the anguish a cancer patient may be feeling.

> I am so afraid. What harsh news. I can't settle down, even though I'm looking upon waves that should be soothing to my soul. Everything I see is colored by the news I received from the doctor. Every aspect of my life is going to change, and oh, I don't want that to happen. Some things I never wanted to change....
>
> Am I fearing death? I don't think so. Not at this point in time. But I am afraid of the future. Of pain. Of the unknown. I have to remember some good could come out of this experience too. That's the way life works....
>
> I think I am afraid of being afraid. What am I going to have to face? I feel so very, very sad.

Sadness, as we know, is not depression. Depression is sadness that cannot find a voice. Depression is encompassing and will not let in any optimism. If the sadness you are feeling continues for more than a few weeks or interferes with your ability to function in your daily tasks, you need to call your doctor. Untreated depression, like cancer, can be life-threatening.

Finding the Right Support Group

Support groups fulfill many needs for people who have cancer. You may feel like you are the only person on earth with your particular problem and that there is no one else who can understand what you are going through right now. Support groups can be a great place for finding others who have "been there, done that" and who are willing to share their experience with you. In a support group you may also find new sources of information about up-to-date medical treatments, strategies to minimize side effects of treatments, and directions for accessing financial assistance.

The most important factor you need to consider when joining a support group is finding one that is appropriate for your needs. Here are some points you should consider before joining one:

Frequency. How often will the group meet? Are the meeting times convenient for you? Is the group a temporary one set up to focus on a single issue or will it meet on an ongoing basis?

Location. Does the group meet in a place that is located nearby and is accessible for you if you have movement limitations? If you won't have access to transportation, you might want to consider joining an online group.

Size. Is the group too large or too small? How intimate do you want the group to be?

Goals. What is the purpose of the group? Does it focus on larger goals, such as education and fund-raising? If it's designed for emotional support, how is the support built into the structure of the group?

Facilitator. Is the group leader a professional or a layperson/peer? You should look for a group that has a good, strong leader who will establish a respectful basis for the exchange of ideas. A well-run group will communicate information to the members via its newsletter or a brochure. If intimate issues might be discussed, the group should have a well-stated confidentiality policy.

Ask your doctors, nurses, or health-care providers for references to support groups. Online resources are available from the American Cancer Society and the National Cancer Institute (see Resources).

Mary's Story

Mary has overcome cancer and has used her experiences to help others form support groups. As she tells people in her group:

"There are times in our lives when we need the support of others to get us through. Whether it comes from family or friends and neighbors, that emotional, spiritual, and physical support is crucial to surviving. And when you are asked to return that support, it is very fulfilling and uplifting to be able to give to others the support and love that were given to you."

Growing up on a farm in southern Minnesota, Mary and her ten siblings learned that if they did not work together with their parents and support each other in doing their chores, the farm would be chaos. When their dad passed away with cancer twenty years earlier and their mom was diagnosed with Alzheimer's two years afterwards, they pulled together and supported each other.

In retrospect, Mary says, "We recognized the value of life, family, and friends, and how important it is to be there for each other."

Their family continued to grow. "Mom and Dad would be very proud of their thirty-two grandchildren and twenty-six great-grandchildren," she says. "Each year on Christmas Day our family rents a hall, because there are more than seventy of us getting together."

But life took a twist for Mary. When she was diagnosed on December 3, 1999, with colorectal cancer at the age of forty-six, the whole family was stunned. She had gone to the doctor thinking she had hemorrhoids but came home with cancer. Her sons, Josh and Tony, had just moved away to college, it was the beginning of the holiday season, work was hectic, and the doctor wanted to start the six-week chemo and radiation treatments immediately to try to shrink the tumor blocking two-thirds of her rectum. The doctor was comforting and reassuring as he explained about the cancer and the processes Mary would be going through, and he did this while also making immediate arrangements for treatment. She knew he was going to take very good care of her, and that helped, but she was concerned about her family.

Woefully, she worried, "How am I going to handle this? How will my family react? What will they say at work? Will I have the support and help I am going to need? Our lives had been disrupted! Chaos!! Who will take care of my family? How is this going to affect my two sons? (They were only eighteen and nineteen and in their first year of college.) And my job—will they allow me to work part-time?"

She continues, "I didn't need to worry. Family, neighbors, and friends rallied around us and took care of everything. Two weeks into treatment, I became very sick and found out I was having an allergic reaction to the chemo. Later I would learn that the radiation had caused an ulcer in the tumor. I was bleeding internally. I couldn't go to work, and by Christmas I'd lost about twenty pounds. When I arrived at the hall on Christmas day, my family reacted first with tears, then hugs and talks, ending with lots of laughs. I knew that no matter what the outcome, I would have all the love and support I needed to deal with this challenge."

Now, five years later, Mary reflects, "Throughout life, the love and support received from family and friends is vitally important. It makes tackling life's challenges so much easier."

Ways You Can Get What You Need from Others

Many excellent lists are available that suggest ways that people can help someone who has cancer. In the back of Brenda Elsagher's book, *If the Battle Is Over, Why Am I Still in Uniform?*, she lists fifty suggestions for friends and family members—from offering to help out with chores, to providing transportation for a family member who needs a car ride, to brightening someone's day with a card or a telephone call. These are all good ideas. Be aware, however, of the roadblocks that may occur when loving, caring friends want to help. One of the barriers hardest to overcome may come from you. The next sections are a discussion of some of those barriers, as well as a few suggestions for getting past them.

Allow Others to Help

As cancer survivors, one of the most difficult things many of us have had to overcome was a reluctance to accept help from others. The vitality I noticed in the survivors I interviewed—the spark that kept them going in the worst of all possible situations—was also what prevented them from allowing others to take over some of their responsibilities.

People who love you will often feel helpless when they see you going through this experience. One of the greatest gifts you can give them is to let them do things for you. Although you may need to hold on to your spirit of independence, it can't hurt to let someone else bring you a meal or do some grocery shopping for you. Letting other people give you rides to your treatments or come over to keep you company when you need a break is not being weak.

You also need to remind caregivers to take good care of themselves. As much as you might need their help, if they run themselves ragged or become run-down, that will only add to your problems. Spreading out the favors you let people do for you is a good way to avoid overloading just a few individuals.

Keep Communication Open

During this time you need to keep an honest exchange of feelings going between you and the people you love to avoid distancing yourselves from each other. Cancer patients often feel isolated, and there's nothing like a good friend who can close that gap.

You may need to assure the people you love that you need to be needed too. They may hesitate to share their daily problems with you, fearing that they will upset you or that their concerns may seem too petty in view of your struggles. Tell them you need to keep involved with their lives too, if that is what you've done in the past. It is very important that the relationships you've enjoyed continue, without a censoring of either person's concerns. If someone's worries become too much of a burden to you, communicate how you're feeling; let them know that, for the present, you have all you can handle just managing your own life.

Another problem that can arise is the difficulty someone on the receiving end might have when you are expressing a negative emotion. Cancer treatments can be the pits. Tiredness and irritability are quite normal reactions, and some side effects, particularly with colorectal cancer, don't make for pleasant topics of conversation. You may need to ask the family member or friend whom you are talking to whether it is all right for you to be frank. You need to express your feelings, but at the same time it's unwise to burden your loved ones with too many complaints. If you feel you are losing perspective, and you have a need to wrestle with dark thoughts more seriously than just talking with a good friend, you should perhaps enlist the help of a counselor or a support group.

Positive Options for Dealing with Your Feelings

◆ Remember that anger, denial, bargaining, and depression are normal, temporary reactions to a diagnosis of colorectal cancer. They may help you cope for a short time. If they persist, seek help. Find a good therapist or someone who cares about you and who will allow you to vent your feelings while helping you get to a better place.

◆ Keep your sense of humor. It will restore your humanity.

◆ Accept the help of your friends and family. Recognize that people will accompany you on this part of the trip in different ways.

◆ Most hospitals offer support groups dealing with all aspects of cancer. Other excellent sources of help can be accessed by visting online resources, such as colon@list serv.acor.org and www.cancer.org.

- Magazines such as *Coping with Cancer* and *Cure* feature inspirational articles and information about all different types of cancer. *Stressfree Living* offers encouraging articles and holistic tips on maintaining good health (see Resources).

- Advocates for Colorectal Education (ACE) is an organization based in Minnesota offering education and nonprofit patient-support programs (see Resources).

Chapter 5

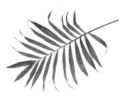

Making Decisions about Treatment

Almost any difficult experience becomes easier to endure through the use of imagery. I remember the fear I felt as I looked out the window of a bus while traveling along the Amalfi Coast in Italy three years ago. Seeing the five hundred-foot drop to the water and the cars racing by on the narrow two-lane highway made me grateful for what I knew about photography. As I framed the pictures with my eyes, "cropping out" all the details I didn't want, my fears decreased and I could focus on the beautiful scenes unfolding before me.

Just like driving along the edge of a five hundred-foot drop, knowing you're headed toward chemotherapy or radiation treatment can dominate your outlook. There may be some moments when you worry that you are about to plunge over a cliff, and others when you find it hard to let the "expert drivers" take over while you ride along as a passenger. At such times the ability to construct a beautiful or peaceful scene in your mind's eye may help you to look beyond the ordeals. It may also pay off to practice your imagery-building skills as another stress-reducing technique.

In addition, education and preparation are good antidotes for feelings of lack of control. Be aware when choosing the right treatment plan for your needs that you have options. Some of these choices include what kind of surgery your doctor is proposing; whether you should undergo radiation, chemotherapy, or both (be sure to learn the pros and cons of all three treatment options); possible treatment schedules; and the side effects you might encounter. Someday, perhaps we will be able to prevent the spread of cancer cells without patients having to endure harsh side effects. Until then, chemotherapy and radiation have been shown to be the most effective means available for destroying these malignant, wayward cells.

Basic Information about Chemotherapy

I discuss chemotherapy in both this chapter and Chapter 8. This chapter focuses on chemotherapy regimens that a patient might undergo *before* surgery for colorectal cancer, and Chapter 8 addresses postsurgical (or adjuvant) chemotherapy treatment.

Chemotherapy involves the use of drugs selected to destroy the cancer cells, which grow more rapidly than other cells. The drugs do their work by attacking the DNA processes of cells while they are growing and reproducing, or dividing. However, for all the good chemotherapy can do, there is a catch, because damage to normal cells also occurs and can result in negative side effects. Chemotherapy may be administered orally or injected into a vein or muscle. It is referred to as a *systemic treatment,* because once the drugs hit the bloodstream, they travel throughout the body. (Of course, the body rebels.)

The detailed treatment plan that your doctor chooses for you to follow is called a treatment *protocol.* Each individual doctor determines his or her protocols. When chemotherapy is used to shrink a tumor before surgery, it is called *neoadjuvant* therapy. When chemotherapy is given after surgery to destroy any cancer cells that may still be present, it is called *adjuvant* therapy. When appropriate, your oncologist may prescribe both therapies—that is, both before and after surgery—or a combination of radiation and chemotherapy.

I asked my friend Kathy Ogle, M.D., an oncologist and writer, what she would like patients to know before beginning chemotherapy. Kathy has a way of cutting through jargon, making complex information clear and easy to understand. Here's what she had to say:

> The word *chemotherapy* is a catchall term that means drug treatment for cancer. There are almost one hundred different drugs used to treat cancer today; some have been in use for decades, and others are brand new.
>
> Every person's cancer situation is different, because every person is different. For most common cancers, however, a standard, or the currently most effective, treatment can be recommended. These recommendations are usually based on the type of cancer, the part of the body it originated in, whether there is sign of its spreading, and how far it has spread. Thus, a person with cancer that began in the colon may receive very different chemotherapy recommendations than a person with cancer that began in the lung. The side effects of chemotherapy vary greatly from one person to another, even among people with the exact same type of cancer who are receiving the exact same chemotherapy. So don't place too much stock in what you have heard from other people about chemotherapy, because the same story may not be at all true for you.
>
> The strength of a chemotherapy treatment can be thought of as lying somewhere on a scale from one to ten. Chemotherapy that is a "one" might be given as a pill, is relatively easy to take, and produces few side effects. Chemotherapy that is a "ten" is probably going to be given in a vein, is expected to be more difficult, and might produce many more side effects. We doctors do not set out with the desire to give harsh treatments. We only use "level-ten" drugs when we have no other choice. In an ideal world, all treatments would be easy and free of side effects, but some cancers only slow down when we treat the patient with our strongest drugs.
>
> Most chemotherapy is given on a specific schedule, with days of treatment and days when there is no treatment. Usually

this is to allow the body's normal tissues to recover and regenerate from side effects. Occasionally, chemotherapy is given every day, most often in the form of a pill.

If you are facing treatment with chemotherapy, the most important thing you can do is to learn as much as possible about your specific type of treatment. Ask lots of questions. Ask for written materials, and take lots of notes. Bring someone with you when the treatment is explained so that a second set of ears can hear what you might miss. Make sure you know how to reach your doctor or a nurse after hours and on weekends, in case you have problems. Find out if there is anything in particular you should be on the lookout for—danger signals that the doctors and nurses need to know about.

In general, the healthier you are before you start chemo, the healthier you will stay throughout the treatments. Keep eating a normal, balanced, healthy diet. Keep exercising as much as your energy will allow. If you are facing chemotherapy, you have had a pretty loud wake-up call about life's unpredictable nature. Take advantage of this opportunity to look forward, look back, and live every minute to its fullest.

And good luck!

Beginning Chemotherapy

The first time you open the door to an oncologist's office, you may feel intimidated, because you probably won't know what to expect. The waiting room most likely will look like any other doctor's office, with patients who might be reading magazines or pleasantly talking with each other. Don't be surprised if you see some of the patients laughing and joking. Humor is one of the main coping mechanisms that cancer survivors cultivate.

Oncologists are accustomed to the fears and misinformation that might burden their patients before treatments, so don't be afraid to ask your doctor for information. Establishing a sense of trust and open communication can be very reassuring.

Some questions you might want to ask your oncologist include the following:

- ◆ What treatments are considered best for my cancer?

- ◆ What kind of a treatment schedule will I be given?

- ◆ What side effects can I expect? What can I do to lessen their impact?

- ◆ Who do I call when I am having difficulty with the treatments? Is there a patient advocate I can talk to?

Common Chemotherapy Treatments

Leucovorin and 5FU (the FU stands for fluorouracil) are two standard drugs currently being prescribed for colorectal cancer treatment. These drugs can be infused into the veins on an outpatient basis using a pump, referred to as a *bolus* procedure, in which the full dosage is given all at once over a short period of time (usually in less than ten minutes). Another method that is gaining popularity is a continuous infusion of 5FU administered through a port (Mediport) implanted under the skin during a minor operation. The port can be refilled with medicine once a week. This method offers the advantage of producing fewer toxic effects. Occasionally, it is necessary to hospitalize the patient for treatment.

Your oncologist will be the one to determine which delivery system, schedule, and medicine are right for you, based on individual factors, such as the location and stage of your cancer, which will have been determined by previous tests. A common schedule for outpatient vein-infusion delivery is either daily doses for five days followed by three weeks off, or once a week for six weeks followed by two weeks off. The most common schedule for drugs continuously infused through a Mediport is to have the medication refilled once a week.

Some Side Effects of Chemotherapy

The American Cancer Society lists the following as the most common side effects of chemotherapy:

- diarrhea

- nausea and vomiting

- loss of appetite

- loss of hair

- mouth sores

- increased chance of infection

- bleeding or bruising after minor cuts or injuries

- fatigue

In addition, you may experience soreness and swelling in the hands and feet, peeling of the skin on the hands and feet, changes in toenails and fingernails, and weight loss. For more information on the side effects of chemotherapy and dealing with them, see "Preparing for the Side Effects of Chemotherapy and Radiation" on page 78 or consult Nancy Bruning's book, *Coping with Chemotherapy.* For more about what worked for me, see "Traveling the Chemotherapy Highway" on page 107.

It is discouraging indeed to view such a grim list, but you need to also keep the following facts in mind:

- Most of the severe side effects of chemotherapy will be short term, diminishing and disappearing after your treatments are over.

- Some people may experience side effects only slightly or not at all. The drugs given for colorectal cancer are usually less devastating than other forms of chemotherapy. Most patients who are given the combination of Leucovorin and 5FU don't lose their hair, though it might thin out temporarily. Nausea, if it occurs, will more than likely be mild.

- Relief for many side effects is available, through medication or alternative healing therapies. Consult your doctor when you are feeling poorly or experiencing pain.

Chemotherapy treatments have a cumulative effect on the body, so the greater the number of treatments you are given, the more you may experience distress. You might feel like you have a mild case of the flu for one or two days after each treatment. Communicate with your oncologist about any difficulties you encounter, as drugs are often available to counteract these problems. Fatigue is common, but many people continue to work if they are able to do so, perhaps on a modified schedule.

An Oncologist Answers Questions about Chemotherapy

My oncologist, Mark D. Sborov, M.D., from the Minnesota Oncology/Hematology Professional Association, recently answered the following questions about scheduling treatments, the effectiveness of treatments in relation to side effects, and clinical trials:

Q: *Why are there different schedules for treatment?*

A: We treat the disease and then we take into account the patient within that disease category. Protocols for chemotherapy are determined by disease. Doses are based upon the drugs used. Within the disease category, sometimes we are blessed with different protocols, and we can pick one based upon the patient's age and underlying medical condition, as long as we can still focus primarily on producing the desired effect.

Q: *How will I know if the treatment is working? What if I have no side effects?*

A: Chemo is not a "no-pain-no-gain" deal. Chemo drugs that are used for specific malignancies will have specific side effects. Sometimes the side effects are significant, like nausea, vomiting, hair loss, and bone-marrow suppression. Some will even have potential side effects on other organs, like the heart and kidneys. Others are relatively benign. The effectiveness of a particular drug is not defined by the side effects it might produce.

Q: *What about clinical trials? Are they only reserved for terminally ill patients?*

A: Clinical trials aren't just for patients with advanced disease. They are available to treat different cancers and at different stages of disease. You might want to participate in a clinical trial for three reasons. First, all of the progress we've made in cancer treatment is because of research. Second, you would have access to treatment that is not otherwise available, and that could benefit you. Third, this is especially true when there are no further conventional treatments available to treat you.

Clinical trials have resulted in the FDA approval of several of the effective chemotherapy treatments currently in use. In each case, cancer patients who participated in the trials received access to the drugs before they became available to the general public. One such drug is Camptostar (CPT11). It is used frequently today in conjunction with 5FU and Leucovorin for stage IV patients. The FDA has recently approved a new drug, Eloxatin, that also works in combination with 5FU and Leucovorin; the combination of the three drugs is called the FOLFOX regime. Xeloda is a drug that has been approved as an oral medicine, and Avastin and Erbitux have been approved by the FDA for the treatment of advanced colorectal cancer. Check with your doctor about side effects.

Researchers are working diligently to find drugs that are the most effective with the fewest side effects. More options exist now for chemotherapy than ever before. Your oncologist can guide you in learning about the newest chemotherapy treatments available and in considering the best regimen for your needs.

Basic Information about Radiation Therapy

Whereas chemotherapy limits cell division, radiation damages the DNA of a cancer cell, thus completely destroying the cell. That's what we want, right? However, the higher the dose of radiation, the greater the number of healthy adjacent cells that are also killed in the process. As with chemotherapy, it's the ultimate trade-off: To destroy cancerous cells, healthy cells are sacrificed.

Thus, when radiation is targeted to a malignant tumor needing treatment, other areas close to the tumor, such as the bladder, sexual organs, or kidney, can also be affected. For this reason, when treating colorectal cancer, radiation is used only for more advanced cases (stages II, III, or IV). Radiation cannot take the place of surgery in effectiveness against the disease, but it is often delivered before rectal surgery to shrink the tumor with the hopes of preserving sphincter muscles.

If your doctors prescribe radiation, you will want answers to essentially the same questions you had about chemotherapy: How often and how long will you be getting treatments, what are the side effects of the treatment, and what are the potential risks versus the benefits?

Treatment by Radiation

Like chemotherapy, radiation treatments can be administered before or after surgery. In addition, radiation therapy is sometimes given during surgery; this is called *intraoperative radiotherapy.*

The standard way of delivering radiation is through *external beam therapy.* During this procedure, high-energy electromagnetic beams radiate the tumor through the skin. The process is quick, lasting approximately fifteen minutes after the patient has been positioned accurately. Schedules for delivering radiation vary, but commonly you will be given daily treatments for five weeks.

Side Effects of Radiation

Radiation is painless when delivered, and most patients do not experience any negative symptoms from early radiation treatments. As with chemotherapy, the side effects of radiation become more pronounced as the dosage accumulates; therefore, the greater the number of treatments, the more intense the side effects.

The most common short-term side effects are the following:

◆ diarrhea/constipation

◆ fatigue

◆ mild skin irritation

◆ rectal or bladder irritation

◆ loss of appetite or nausea

◆ decreased white blood cell count

◆ mouth sores caused by stomach upsets

Potential Long-Term Risks and Benefits

The above symptoms more than likely will disappear as soon as treatments are over. However, some people experience substantial and more permanent side effects from radiation.

As mentioned above, neighboring organs that fall into the field of radiation may be the most affected. Radiation treatment for colorectal cancer can be responsible for damage to reproductive organs in both males and females. This can result in decreased ejaculate and retrograde ejaculation in men and early menopause in women. It can also cause some degree of permanent bladder or rectal irritation.

Infrequently, radiation can cause *radiation proctitis,* an inflammation in the lining of the rectum. Radiation proctitis can occur at any time, from months to years after a patient has completed the radiation therapy. Although the problem is usually short-lived, it can become a chronic, long-term problem in up to 15 percent of patients, resulting in a possible discharge of blood or mucus from the rectum.

Our ACE group asked Amy Thorsen, M.D., from Colon and Rectal Associates, the following question:

Q: *If someone is given radiation treatment for colorectal cancer, would that affect his or her ability to have children?*

A: Radiation therapy for rectal cancer can interfere with gonadal (ovarian and testicular) function, leading to temporary or permanent infertility. Women with a history of pelvic radiation who get pregnant are at risk for low-birth-weight neonates (newborns). Radiation can also lead to erectile dysfunction in men. Chemotherapy can cause premature ovarian failure in women, leading to infertility. Because both chemotherapy and radiation cause potential toxicity, pregnancy should be avoided when either partner is receiving treatment.

Again, side effects vary with each individual. Because of the potential risk of infertility, if this is an issue for you, you may want to consider banking ova or sperm for the future before undergoing radiation therapy or chemotherapy. Women may want to explore the option of using hormone replacement therapies or local estrogen creams for vaginal dryness.

The damage done by radiation often declines with time, and, in spite of the risks, radiation therapy can produce significant benefits for colorectal cancer patients. It can save the sphincter muscles by decreasing the size of the tumor before surgery. It has been shown to enhance the effectiveness of chemotherapy, and in cases where surgery is not possible, it can increase chances of survival and can offer palliative benefits (benefits that lessen the severity of the disease's symptoms). As would be the case with any exposure to radiation, possible sterilization of reproductive organs and damage to neighboring tissues are risks that should not be taken lightly. These are important issues to discuss with your doctor and perhaps a patient advocate.

Paul's Story

Paul Leland, age forty-one, was the head accountant for a public corporation. While undergoing a flexible sigmoidoscopy, he received the unfortunate news from his gastrologist that there was a high probability he had rectal cancer. He was given what he describes as a "whirlwind tour" of every conceivable test before he was diagnosed with stage II colorectal cancer.

Before surgery, he underwent a radiation schedule of five straight weeks in combination with chemotherapy delivered by continuous infusion. As the technicians measured Paul for a semipermanent tattoo [to mark where the radiation should be delivered], he thought to himself with a wry sense of humor, "I sure hope they know what they're doing." As a mathematician as well as a patient, he knew the importance of getting the measurements right.

Paul tends to downplay his ordeals as he recounts them today, but he experienced mouth sores, diarrhea, nausea, and fatigue. Nevertheless, he was able to keep working, which he believes was helpful. About three weeks after he completed the presurgery treatments, the short-term side effects gradually disappeared.

"I did what I had to do," Paul remembers. "Although deep down I was frightened and saddened that I had rectal cancer, I was well grounded in my faith and my trust in my doctors. With the help of my family, I got by."

Four years later, even though the longer-term effects of radiation and surgery continue to present him with challenges to his digestive system, Paul is making an excellent recovery from his bout with colorectal cancer. He advises new cancer patients to "ask a lot of questions and help develop your own treatment plan."

Myths about Radiation Therapy

Certain false conceptions exist about radiation. One of the most prevalent is that a radiation patient becomes radioactive. What actually happens is that the radiant energy is converted into a biochemical agent that injures or destroys the DNA of selected cells. Another myth is that radiation is harmless. People react differently to radiation, just as people react differently to the sun's rays. Although the risks of the side effects of radiation are less than the benefits gained by killing the cancer cells, keep in mind that radiation is a powerful treatment. Ask about all the possible side effects that might affect you as an individual, and realize that you can put a stop to treatment when you feel you have had enough.

As discussed throughout this chapter, treatment of colorectal cancer with high dosages of radiation can damage reproductive organs and cause sterility, among other long-term effects.

My Experience with Radiation Therapy

Radiation can be administered in a number of ways. My treatment was to be delivered through my skin, by external beam therapy. When I walked into the radiation room, my first thought was "You've got to be kidding." The room reminded me of a movie set

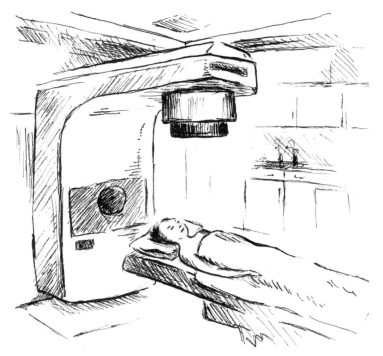

Figure 3. External beam therapy.

from a 1950s sci-fi drama where the heroine was about to be transported to some distant planet. It was darkened, and before me was a gigantic white-plastic beamer approximately twenty-feet tall (see Figure 3).

I was told to remove all clothes from the waist down, climb onto a footstool, and lie facedown under the X-ray machine. In a test run, the exact area where I was to be radiated was pinpointed and marked on my left buttock with a painless temporary tattoo with semipermanent ink. I was told the tattoo would withstand bathing but not rubbing, and would remain for the whole six weeks. The technicians were required to leave me alone in the room during my treatments so that they were not unnecessarily exposed to high levels of radiation. That should have told me something. They assured me they would be monitoring the whole process and that it would last just a few minutes.

I was lying face down, but I could hear the whirring of the machine as it beamed radiation down on the chosen spot in my anal area. I was told to breathe normally and not move. I tried to avoid letting my imagination convince me I was going to be transported to Mars. Instead, I started to fantasize I was in a microwave oven being nuked with rays. That thought terrified me, so I switched to imagining I was in a tanning booth getting bronzed. That image worked for me.

Before I knew it, the procedure was over. I had been given a special parking stamp allowing me to pull right up to the curb in front of the door to the radiation department. I went home pleased with the way I had faced up to all I had encountered that first day and relieved it was over.

Being diagnosed with stage III rectal cancer, I was given three preoperative chemotherapy treatments. I experienced only mild feelings of nausea and proceeded over the next two weeks to drive myself to the hospital for radiation treatments every day after work, hop onto the table, receive my "tanning session," and return home. For the first two weeks I wondered what all the fuss was about. I didn't suffer much reaction to the chemotherapy treatments, and I wasn't getting any reaction from the radiation. In fact, I was joking about my "tanning booth."

My life took on a predictable pattern. Every day at 3:00 P.M., when I finished teaching school, I would drive to the hospital, park in a spot reserved for radiation patients, go in, and get "zapped." I became very agile at performing this routine, and the nurses kidded that I was setting records for getting on and off the table quickly. During my treatments I would imagine a beautiful scene, such as the water lapping on the rocks of Lake Superior, and think of myself lying there enjoying the sunshine.

Those first weeks were a time of self-indulgence and euphoria. I ate whatever I felt like eating. Now that I was done with the first dosages of chemo and actually receiving radiation, it was so painless I felt rather free of fear. People went out of their way to be kind to me, and I was particularly kind to myself. While waiting in traffic during the daily drive to my radiation treatments, I played the soundtrack to *Lord of the Dance* and Andrea Bocelli's *Romanza* over and over. The sunrises greeted me each morning with their pearl-like charm. I wore an Irish Claddaugh ring for luck.

By the third week, I was still free from many side effects. I was even questioning my decision not to return to work after vacation was over. The only trouble I was having was a loss of appetite. Gradually, without realizing it, I was also cutting down on fluid intake. Not a good thing to do! I experienced some gastric upsets and took medication for diarrhea almost daily. Every day, to minimize the effects of radiation, I was supposed to take sitz baths at home (sit in a tub filled with a few inches of warm water). Still trying to infuse some pleasure into the situation, I pretended that I was at a spa, and I filled the bathroom with candles as I lay soaking in the bathtub.

By the fourth week, the scene changed. I was nauseated quite often and extremely tired all the time. I did not know about the devastating effects dehydration could have on the body and wasn't aware that my lack of fluid intake was probably causing additional problems. (See Chapter 8 for more about the importance of maintaining adequate fluid intake during radiation and chemotherapy.) Since I'm a redhead, my skin was more than usually sensitive to the strong dosages of radiation I was receiving. I ended up with bladder and urinary infections that caused me quite a bit of short-term discomfort. And five years later, I am still plagued with symptoms of radiation proctitis. In retrospect, it would have been a good idea for me to exercise my option of stopping the treatments a few days short of the full five weeks. Doing so may have lessened the damage to my neighboring tissues. At the time, however, I did not realize I had the option of stopping treatments whenever I felt that doing so was necessary or would be helpful.

Preparing for the Side Effects of Chemotherapy and Radiation

The book *Radiation and Chemotherapy for Cancer: Mind-Body Therapy for Healing,* by Alene Christiano, Ed.D., is entirely devoted to the ways in which patients can prepare themselves for the challenges of dealing with side effects. The author takes a holistic approach to healing and is a strong advocate of nurturing the immune system while going through radiation and chemotherapy. Dr. Christiano advises patients to

1. learn what they need to know

2. prepare for the worst

3. expect the best

Preparation is the key here, yet she also encourages patients to expect to be in the group that will experience the least amount of trouble. Focusing on the positive aspects of what the treatments are trying to do, she believes, will help patients see this period of time as temporary, and the benefits as permanent.

What sorts of things does Dr. Christiano mean by "preparation"? Affirmations and visualization, finding ways to nurture the soul and the body, prayer, meditation, relaxation, massage, and eliminating unnecessary stress are good preparations for anyone who is encountering a difficult challenge. Eating well, getting plenty of rest, and exercising will strengthen the immune system, and are also generally good ideas for maintaining overall health.

Good nutrition is a must. Make an appointment to consult with a dietician about your needs.

As mentioned earlier, mouth sores can be a common but agonizing side effect. Salivary gland dysfunction can lead to drymouth. This condition can foster tooth decay and resultant sores, which can be so painful that they may require hospitalization or disrupt treatments. It is highly recommended that you visit your dentist before beginning any cancer therapy. A good cleaning with a fluoride treatment can possibly save you much grief. Using a 1.01 percent sodium fluoride dentifrice prescribed by your dentist could reduce infections. A nonalcoholic mouthwash will help to keep your mouth from becoming too dry. You can also keep your mouth moist by sucking ice chips and drinking lots of water. Keep flossing your teeth gently, and switch to an extra-soft or child's toothbrush for daily brushing.

Most colorectal patients do not lose their hair, but it can happen. If you want to be prepared, you could be fitted before hair loss occurs, while your hair is still in its natural state and color.

As mentioned in the last chapter, when people make offers to help, accept them. As insurance against getting caught with no transportation to a treatment appointment, put together a list of people whom you could call if you need a ride—or if you need to take them up on their generosity in other ways.

Questionable Treatments

When you are facing treatments for colorectal cancer, it's important to realize how vulnerable you are. It's tempting to be talked into therapies that make promises you want to hear: the promise of a quick fix without harmful side effects. Good information can be found in the *Guide to Complementary and Alternative Cancer Methods*, a pamphlet published by the American Cancer Society, and on the National Cancer Institute's Medline website at www.medlineplus.org. You should also visit the Quackwatch website at www.quackwatch.org. The site makes a distinction between genuine alternatives, which have met the criteria for safety and effectiveness, and questionable alternatives, which are unproven and lack scientific basis. Other websites also exist that can answer questions about alternative therapies (see Resources, located in the back of this book).

The American Cancer Society evaluates therapies for cancer by asking the following three questions:

1. Is the method objective and has it been demonstrated through peer-reviewed literature to be effective?

2. Does the method offer potential benefits that will outweigh the negative side effects?

3. Have studies on the method been carefully conducted, with appropriate peer review?

Other questions to consider include the following:

◆ How much money will the treatment cost?

◆ What does your doctor think about this method or product?

◆ Is there compatibility between the use of this alternative and your conventional plan of healing?

◆ What are the experts' credentials?

In addition, look at the way the therapy is being sold. Advertising that makes extremely paranoid statements about the government, the FDA, and your doctors should send up a red flag about the legitimacy of the product. Pseudomedical jargon and anecdotal testimonials, especially in place of bona fide research, should be viewed with suspicion. The National Cancer Institute strongly recommends that patients consult a qualified, board-certified doctor before spending money on questionable forms of treatment.

Promoters of these treatments often fill books with testimonials from people claiming "cures" but at the same time cannot prove what they say with research. The danger here is that patients can lose valuable time and thus the opportunity to undergo potentially effective therapy that could result in a cure or better control of the disease.

Complementary therapies do exist that offer enormous relief for patients looking for stress reduction, improvement in quality of life, and to combat the harsh effects of chemotherapy and radiation. For a discussion of some of these, see the section in Chapter 7 titled "Steps to Healing: Being Helped by Complementary Therapies." At the same time, be aware that a treatment may not be harmless just because it is described as "natural." Some homeopathic medicines and dietary supplements may, in fact, react negatively with certain chemotherapy treatments. It is important to talk with your doctors when considering any supplementary care. In addition, evaluate practitioners of any therapy with regard to their training, their credentials, and the financial gain they would realize if you were to buy their products or services.

Positive Options for Making Decisions about Treatments

♦ Research the potential side effects of each cancer treatment before you see the doctor.

♦ Ask questions. You have the right to be informed. If you are experiencing pain or are worried about the possible outcomes of your treatment, consult a doctor who will listen to you. Remember, you have the right to decide how much you are willing to endure with regard to harsh side effects.

♦ Dehydration can become a problem. Take seriously the suggestion that you should drink at least eight glasses of water a day.

♦ Make sure you are getting adequate nutrition in your diet. Supplemental vitamins and minerals may be helpful, but consult your doctor before taking extremely high doses of any substance—even vitamins and minerals. Some supplements can interact adversely with medical treatments.

◆ Consult your dentist about measures for preventing mouth sores. A fluoride treatment and use of a nonalcoholic mouthwash may help. Keep your mouth moist by sucking on ice chips.

◆ Sitz baths and aloe-based lotions approved by your doctor are helpful for the dry skin that may result from radiation treatments.

◆ Meditate or create beautiful pictures in your mind. Do whatever is relaxing and therapeutic. Keep practicing the breathing technique you learned in Chapter 1.

◆ Before trying any alternative treatments for cancer, evaluate them based on their known effectiveness, their benefits, and the validity of any studies that have tested them. Consult with your medical team before undergoing any complementary treatments.

Chapter 6

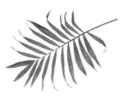

Coping with Surgery: Plain Talk about a Complicated Subject

Cancer cells have no manners. They barge in uninvited and respect no boundaries. Eventually, if left to themselves, they spread to other areas of the body, causing mortal harm. Ignoring them won't help; they'll just gang up on you.

When Is Surgery Necessary?

Almost all colorectal cancers begin with a harmless-looking polyp that resembles a small grape. Generally speaking, the larger the polyp, the greater the chance of it being cancerous. Thirty to 50 percent of all polyps in the colon are of a type called *adenomatous polyps*. If left alone, adenomatous polyps have a great chance of developing into cancer. Think of them as cancer "wannabes." The only way to be sure they won't become dangerous is to get them out of there, and that requires surgery.

Unless the polyps are so large that they are blocking your intestines, you can usually delay your surgery for several weeks. Colorectal cancers tend to be slow-growing; taking a few weeks before surgery often won't make much difference and might give you time to catch your breath. You may need to make special arrangements for yourself or your family.

The primary goal of surgery for colorectal cancer is to remove as much of the malignant tumor as possible, while causing the least amount of damage. Very early cancers can be removed during an examination with a sigmoidoscope or during a colonoscopy. In this case, if the polyp is completely removed, no further treatments are necessary, other than keeping a watchful eye on the colon.

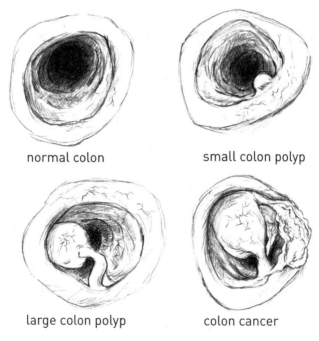

normal colon   small colon polyp

large colon polyp   colon cancer

Figure 4. Noncancerous and cancerous polyps.

For early stages of rectal cancer in particular, a less invasive operation called a *local excision* may be an option. A local excision can be done on an outpatient basis by removing the polyp through the anus. Further treatment will depend on the depth of invasion by the cancer cells into the moist lining of the muscle wall (the mucosa). [See Figure 2 on page 27 and Figure 4 above.]

In cases where there is some question as to whether or not the polyp has been completely removed, further surgery is usually required. Any part of a polyp that has been left behind could turn out to contain malignant cells. Surgery is especially recommended for polyps containing malignant cells that are in danger of spreading to lymph nodes. The location and the staging of the tumor will determine what kind of surgery is needed. The most accurate way to stage a tumor is by removing local lymph nodes and studying them under a microscope. The surgeon will examine the pelvic area, abdomen, and liver to determine the spread of the cancer.

Most cases in which the cancer has spread will require a *resection*, a procedure in which portions of the intestine (bowel) are removed through an incision in the lower abdomen. The remaining ends are then reattached to each other using a process called *anastomosis*. Remember, most of your food is digested before it reaches the colon, so you can function quite well even if part of the colon is removed and reattached. Most resections today use special staples that can be taken out seven to ten days after surgery. Some of the tissue surrounding the diseased portion of the bowel, as well as neighboring lymph nodes, will also be removed. Samples of the removed tissue will be sent to a pathology lab for testing. The pathologist will send a report back to your doctor, who will make recommendations for further treatment based on this evidence.

You have the option to request that the hospital preserve a sample from your tumor on a slide once it has been surgically removed and to keep it in a bank. This sample would be good to have if you want to be genetically tested or if a recurrence should occur.

Every effort will be made to save your sphincter muscles. However, if you have rectal cancer, you may face additional problems. Rectal surgery is technically more difficult and complex than colon surgery. The rectum has a different function than the colon; it is the rectum that stores bodily wastes. You may be able to have an operation that will save your sphincter muscles, called a *lower anterior resection*. In this situation, your surgeon may recommend that you receive a temporary, diverting ostomy. An *ostomy* is a surgically created opening in the abdomen through which undigested food (waste matter) can pass into a bag, where it is stored until you are ready to empty it. Part of the intestine is brought to the body's surface to make the new opening. This is called a *stoma*. See the next section for more about stomas and temporary ostomies.

If too much of the rectum has to be removed, you may need to have a permanent ostomy. See Chapter 9 for more about permanent ostomies.

Temporary Ostomies

When I was talking with Dr. Nemer, my colorectal surgeon, about planning for my treatments and resection surgery, he delivered a zinger. I would have to have a temporary ileostomy for at least six weeks following surgery.

"A what?" I asked.

"It's like a bypass of your digestive system. An opening in your abdominal wall. It will allow you to heal."

"Are you talking about a bag?" I had heard whispers about those. At this point, my vanity took over. Even with all the other, more hazardous kinds of treatment we had discussed, this one bothered me the most by far. I wanted no more of this conversation, and I started to consider that maybe I would just hide my head in the sand and forget the whole thing.

He had obviously encountered this kind of resistance before, and he was ready for it. "It's probably going to be temporary, remember that," he repeated. "Most patients don't need a permanent ostomy. If everything goes according to plan, we will reverse the operation in six weeks." He suggested that I schedule a visit with the enterostomal nurses at Fairview Hospital, Vicki Haugen and Julie Powell.

In eight days I would start treatments in chemotherapy and radiation. In about eight weeks I would be scheduled for surgery. Still, all I could think about was the ileostomy, and I was resistant. I had not bargained for it.

First Aid: The Enterostomal Nurses

Despite my antagonistic feelings about the proposed ostomy, I made an appointment with the enterostomal nurses. I knew that to refuse to undergo the resection would be too risky. I realized the importance of taking immediate action, and getting a temporary ostomy was going to be part of the ordeal. I reluctantly decided to at least get more information.

When I met with Vicki Haugen, she didn't try to pretend that my needing to have an ostomy was good news. "Let me tell you what this is all about," she said. I was ready to listen. Actually, I was curious.

She led me into an examining room filled with charts and supplies and showed me a detailed chart of the colon and the upper part of the small intestine. It was one of the best maps of the human digestive system I have seen. (By then I had become somewhat of a connoisseur of digestive drawings.) We zeroed in on the picture of the small intestine. It's about twenty feet long and is coiled loosely in the abdomen.

After resection surgery, different types of ostomies are performed, depending on how much and what part of the intestine is removed. If the tumor is low in the rectum and the surgeon can't resect above it, the patient usually gets a *colostomy,* an ostomy located in the sigmoid colon, the lowest part of the colon (see Figure 6 on page 121). If the tumor is higher, the surgeon may resect the tumor and give the patient an *ileostomy,* an ostomy located in the ileum, the end of the lowest part of the small intestine, enabling the colon and the new resected area to heal for a while before they are reconnected. It is rare, but sometimes a colostomy or an ileostomy may need to be permanent, depending on many factors. Usually, though, the ostomy is temporary.

As mentioned earlier, the place where the intestine is brought out to the outer abdominal wall is called a stoma. It is reddish-pink in color, sort of like the inside of your mouth. There is no valve to shut it off. In my case, the ileum would be brought out of my abdominal wall. Digestive material would pass through my body, out through my stoma, and into a pouch on a continuous basis. I would have to wear the pouch as long as I had the ostomy.

When I heard this, I must have grimaced. Vicki picked up on my reaction and kept reassuring me to stay with her as she explained the rest. She then showed me the first picture I had ever seen of a stoma. It was so small and so unprotected; it could hardly take on the role of the ugly monster I had pictured in my mind. The bags she showed me, which I had so strongly set my mind against, were the size of a small sandwich bag. They were disposable, white, would be attached by an adhesive to my skin, and would be completely sanitary.

But what of the reality of having to wear the bag all the time? Would there be an odor when I was in public? What kind of clothes would I have to wear?

Vicki assured me that when I was with other people, no one would have to be aware I was wearing an appliance. However, dressing in clingy spandex shorts was probably out. (I replied that, at my age, it was out for me anyway.) The idea that no one would ever have to know appealed to me. I could keep my secret buried forever. Vicki reassured me that the new disposable bags were efficient and odor-free. Emptying them regularly would prevent telltale bulges, and using a small amount of water while doing this would make the process more efficient.

I got the clear message that having an ostomy would be as bad or as good as I made it. The adjustment was up to me. Although Vicki was not minimizing my concerns, she was certainly helping to take the sting out of them.

The other enterostomal nurse, Julie, came in to see how everything was going, and the three of us talked a bit about my colorectal surgeon. Their positive comments reaffirmed my feelings of confidence in him; they also readily endorsed the oncologist and the radiation specialist who had been recommended to me.

I left their office feeling hopeful. I was surprised at the turnaround in my attitude. Now I was feeling "lucky." Not lucky that I had cancer, certainly. Nor that I had to have an ileostomy. But if I was going to have to take such a journey, I felt I had been placed on a superhighway lined with competent and helpful caregivers. I would not be abandoned on a lonely road. People who I felt were trustworthy were taking my hand, leading the way to a safer place. Enterostomal nurses do so much more than just giving out medical advice. They are in a strategic position to guide patients who feel incredibly lost.

Suggestions for Your Hospital Stay

Jan Gray, in the "Senior's Corner" column she writes for the Minneapolis-area *Sun* newspaper, published a list of practical suggestions for patients to consider before going into the hospital, to make the process less stressful. When I interviewed Jan, a member of ACE, I asked her, "What turned out to be the most helpful tip you used during your hospital stay?" Jan replied, "Use your voice mail or answering machine to best advantage by changing your message to inform people that you will be in the hospital. Let them leave you their best wishes, and when you are out of recovery you can access the messages from the hospital phone. That saves you from talking to each person individually at a time when you are least able to do so, and yet you can still have those wonderful caregiving messages coming in. Also, if you establish a telephone tree, then your family members only need to call one or two people to let others know the latest update on your recovery."

The following are Jan's other suggestions:

- Ask the physician about the risks and benefits of the procedure before the operation, and inquire what choices of hospitals you have. Some might be more convenient for you than others.

- Call your insurance company. Be sure the operation is preapproved.

- Check with your doctor for preoperative instructions.

◆ Find out which medications you should or should not be taking. For example, drugs that thin the blood, such as aspirin or ibuprofen, should not be taken for at least two weeks before surgery.

◆ Follow all instructions about drinking fluids and eating before surgery. Neglecting to do this may even postpone your surgery.

◆ Decide whether you will have a health-care directive, power of attorney, or patient's bill of rights filled out and on file before you enter surgery. These documents are designed to secure your wishes if life-saving interventions are necessary. For example, some people, for religious reasons, may object to receiving a transfusion. You need to initiate a discussion of these issues if your health-care team does not bring them up.

◆ Finally, you may need to arrange care for yourself after hospitalization.

What Should You Take to the Hospital?

Clothing. It's not a fashion show, but still, you may have company after your first few days. The hospital will supply gowns and robes, but you may want to cover them with a bed-jacket or a nightshirt. In the beginning, you will be hooked up to intravenous equipment, so you need to wear something that has loose sleeves and that opens in the front for convenience. Thick sports socks may come in handy while you're lying in bed. Slippers will be supplied by the hospital, but you'll probably be charged for them.

Toiletries. Bring your own shampoo, toothpaste, and deodorant. Razors should be disposable or battery-operated. Women should also bring feminine products and makeup (if they normally wear it). And since you will have to remove your nail polish before surgery, you may want to bring some so you can reapply it after you have fully recovered from the anesthesia.

Extras. Bring your eyeglasses or contact lenses for use after you recover from surgery. Bring along a *TV Guide* for the week and crossword puzzles from the paper that you didn't have time to finish before you left home. Now is the time to catch up on the reading you always wanted to do, so bring along a good book. Hospitals can be bright and noisy, so pack eye coverings and/or earplugs to help you sleep. Pack photos you want to keep with you as well as phone numbers of close friends and a calling card for making long-distance calls.

If you enjoy a particular kind of music, you may want to bring a Walkman so you can play it when you want to. If you use headphones, you won't annoy your roommate when you turn up the volume. You might want to bring your own pillow if it will help you to sleep better. Notecards with addresses are helpful if you decide to catch up on your correspondence.

Money. You won't feel much like going on a shopping spree, but you might want to bring a small amount of loose change for newspapers, snacks, etc.

Your sense of humor. This may sound contrary to everything you feel right now, but most patients agree that a good laugh can be very therapeutic. Scott Burton, a cancer survivor, comedian, and author of *A Life in Balance,* has this to say: "It's important to remember that there is not and never will be anything funny about cancer—which is why some feel they can't, or shouldn't, laugh. But what is funny is life. It always has been. From your first greeting in the world being a smack on the bottom to the fact that time will eventually turn you into your parents, life is a wondrous comedy. In dealing with cancer, life is different, but it's not any less present. So, just as there was humor in life before cancer, there can be humor in life during cancer."

Marcia, an ACE member, has a delightful story about this:

Marcia's Story

Following my diagnosis, I did a lot of things to get ready for my surgery. I remembered Norman Cousins' theory that laughter heals [he wrote the book *Anatomy of an Illness*]. One of the things I did was to call a comedy club and explain that I needed a comedian to come and see me after surgery. The club connected me to a cancer survivor and comedian named Scott Burton, who offered to visit me in the hospital. The night before he was scheduled to come to the hospital, my brother, sister-in-law, niece, and two friends showed up for a visit. They were very funny that night, and we were all in stitches. We were laughing so hard, I was surprised they didn't throw us out. I was actually holding my side because it hurt from laughing. I said to them, "What are you doing to me?" It was one of those rare occasions; I'll never forget it. The next day I called Scott and told him I was doing okay and he didn't need to come; that my family had already succeeded in making me laugh. He told me, "Take care. If you change your mind, you can always call me." Although I never met him face-to-face, that meant a lot to me.

The Operating Room

From the perspective of being the one on the table, being in an operating room is an almost surreal experience. When it was my turn, I found myself looking up at white acoustic ceiling panels and glaring lights, surrounded by pale ceramic walls that were more like what I would expect to see in a bathroom rather than in a place where surgery was going to happen. People in the room were at an angle that made them appear elongated and as though they were floating in space. They were preparing to look around in my body, and just for a moment I was not sure I was going to give them permission to do that. Then I heard the commanding voice of Dr. Nemer, my colorectal surgeon. As he looked down to greet me, he asked, "Are you ready?"

I nodded. I knew at that minute I was going to cooperate as much as I could. Actually, the word *co-operate* is wonderfully descriptive of that moment. I became part of the operating team and said a silent prayer as the anesthesiologist put me to sleep. I thought to myself, "This has to be the epitome of trust"… and then all was oblivion.

For the next twenty-four hours I can't remember being in pain. I must have been, of course, considering that six inches of my rectum had been removed, but I can't remember it. I was well attended to and kept warm. I was even coaxed into getting up and walking the next day.

Length of hospital stays vary, but you can expect to be there for at least five to six days. Most patients are on strong pain medication for a minimum of three days. You must make it clear to your nurses when you are experiencing pain, as too much pain can interfere with your healing. You can expect to be asked to rate your pain on a scale from one to ten. The nurse will explain to you specifically what that means. Gradually, you will be weaned off morphine through the use of a patient-controlled infusion pump that will administer medication only when you need it. You need not worry about overdosing; the device won't let you do that.

The Recovery Room

Hearing is one of the first senses to return when you are in recovery. You start to hear even before your eyes start to open, and people around you should be careful of what they are saying long before you begin to look like you are awake. Ruth's story shows why.

Ruth's Story

When Ruth was in the recovery room regaining consciousness after her surgery, she looked like she was still asleep. She remembers someone in the room talking about the fact that she needed to have a biopsy on her liver. The remark registered. This is not the time for a patient to learn that she or he is in stage IV of the disease.

Ruth returned to surgery two months later to have a tumor on her liver removed. She remembers that, in spite of the news being dire, she was resolved to live through the experience. When her surgeon came into her room he exclaimed, "Congratulations! There was only one tumor on your liver! You just made my day!"

Ruth responded, "Doctor, you just made my life!"

♪ ♪ ♪

There is no doubt that a diagnosis of cancer is frightening, and having it metastasize to another organ makes it even more threatening. Yet successful surgery can increase a patient's chances of surviving and thriving, even in the case of an advanced cancer. Even when only 20 percent of a person's liver remains, for example, the rest of the liver can regenerate and grow in a healthy way.

As Ruth's liver regenerated following tumor removal, she remembers having nightmares in which she watched her liver grow uncontrollably until it took over her entire being. She once asked her surgeon, "How does it know when to stop?" She was relieved to find out that it does, through some mysterious primal wisdom of the human body.

Positive Options for Coping with Surgery

- Read and follow all directions while preparing for surgery.

- Remember that optimism, a willingness to cooperate and, for those who believe in it, the power of prayer may contribute to the success of your surgery. Fear and negativity may work against the process.

- Restrict early visitors and phone calls. Give yourself time to heal. Use your home answering machine to receive get-well messages.

- Bring supplementary supplies to the hospital to make your stay as comfortable as possible.

- Be sure to communicate your needs and concerns to the doctors and nurses around you. They are there to help.

◆ Talk to your health-care providers about getting patient support, such as having a cancer survivor contact you. Resources for cancer support are listed in the back of this book.

◆ If you will be getting an ostomy, call the United Ostomy Association (UOA) chapter nearest to you. It will send you information and provide you with a visitor, if you so desire. You may also want to read Dr. Craig A. White's book, *Positive Options for Living with Your Ostomy* (see Resources).

Chapter 7

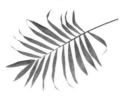

The First Six Weeks
after Surgery

One of the frustrations of having cancer surgery is the lack of information available to tell you what to expect when you come home from the hospital. There is the customary sheet of directions, of course, handed to you as you are being whisked by wheelchair out to an awaiting car. Read it carefully and don't be afraid to ask any questions about directions you don't quite understand.

In addition, talk to your doctors and nurses about postoperative guidelines *before* you leave the hospital. Be sure you have an appointment to see your surgeon soon after you have been discharged from the hospital. You will probably be given the name of a home-health-care agency in case you need assistance once you are at home. Your surgeon or a nurse should explain all medications you need to take and give you a number you can call in case of an emergency.

What to Expect Once You're Home

Once you are home, you may find yourself facing two to six weeks of recovery without many blueprints to tell you if you are recovering according to expectations. This section offers some general guidelines.

Physical Activities

After five to seven days in the hospital, you've probably spent quite a bit of time in bed. Once you are home and resume normal activities, you will feel much more tired than usual. Give yourself plenty of rest breaks to slowly build up your strength. Walking is excellent exercise and can be done for short distances several times a day. You can gradually increase the amount you walk every day. You can climb stairs or do chores around the house that do not involve any lifting.

Almost anything that strains your stomach muscles will work against your healing at this point. Lifting anything more than twenty pounds is unwise and, in fact, may even cause a hernia. It is unwise to operate machinery or drive while under the influence of any narcotic pain medication.

Unless there is some problem, you can usually shower, even with an ostomy. At all other times, you will want to keep your incision clean and dry. To prevent infection, you should probably avoid baths or swimming for at least two weeks after surgery.

Diet

You can gradually resume a normal diet, unless otherwise directed. If you have an ostomy, then the rules change. Consult with your enterostomal nurses about your diet. At the beginning, you will probably be advised to avoid fibrous foods and ease back into an appropriate diet. Nutrition is important, regardless. Eating pureed foods, even foods prepared for babies, might be a good thing to do at the beginning. Be sure to drink plenty of water—a must for all patients, but especially for those with ostomies.

How You Will Feel

It is normal for your incision to look discolored and mildly bruised after surgery. This should resolve itself within twenty-one days.

Your appetite may not be at its best, and you may notice slight changes in your bowel functions for a while, such as diarrhea or constipation. If you have had rectal surgery, you may experience phantom pains, similar to those reported by amputees who have had a limb removed. You may also pass some mucus. You might want to try sitting on the toilet for some time each day, as if you were evacuating your bowel. This sometimes will relieve the discomfort you are feeling.

When You Need to Call Your Doctor

Call your doctor if you notice any of the following symptoms:

* if bleeding, pain, or drainage occurs near your incision
* if your temperature is over 101°F or is consistently above average
* if you experience abdominal pain that is not relieved by medication
* if you experience excessive discomfort with constipation, diarrhea, or bloating, or your problems last for more than a few days
* if you have other concerns about your health

Above all, it's good advice to relax and to take your recovery one day at a time. Listen to your body and pace yourself.

❦ ❦ ❦

When I came home from the hospital, I went through a period of elation, a quiet stillness that only someone worn down by the strife of reconstruction can appreciate. It was a relief from the onslaught of harsh treatments and a newly acquired appreciation of the ordinary rituals of life—awakening to a day free from doctor appointments and hospital schedules, relishing the taste of food again, focusing on concerns other than disease.

My first week after returning home was a blur. I was well supplied with pain pills and glad to get out of the hospital. I took time to look out at our trees in the backyard and marveled that we were already in the last weeks of May. By the second week, the pain pills were wreaking havoc on my stomach, and I decided it was time to stop taking them. I would occasionally wake up in the middle of the night, anxious and still sore from the operation. I switched to Tylenol and sleeping pills for a few days, and then decided I could get by just taking the Tylenol. Everyone is different in this regard, however. Cards, phone calls, and visits from friends kept me in good spirits.

The stitches in my abdomen were healing nicely, and the new ostomy wasn't giving me any problems. I thought of the ostomy as a minor impediment in my recovery, a small detour while my main thoroughfare was being repaired. However, by the end of the fourth week after surgery, I was surprised that I was still experiencing so much rectal discomfort. I couldn't be on my feet for more than twenty minutes without hurting. I had to lie down in the backseat of the car if we were going to ride for more than an hour. I felt phantom pains that gave me the urge to evacuate. I didn't know that these problems were in the normal range and would soon begin to fade. Healing is a work in progress.

Follow-Up to Surgery

You need to be conscientious about cooperating with the follow-up plan your health-care team has developed. Blood tests, colonoscopies, endoscopies, and other tests are necessary to identify possible recurrences. Rectal ultrasounds are recommended for patients with rectal cancer. CEA tests can be helpful in detecting cancer and are usually part of a follow-up plan.

Protocols vary, but your surgeon will map out a schedule for your visits. Usually, you will see some medical specialist every three months for two years, and thereafter every six months for another three years. After five years of good results, colorectal cancer patients are considered "cured"; however, they remain at a higher degree of risk for developing colorectal cancer in the future.

Special Problems

Following surgery, particularly surgery in the small intestine, adhesions may form. These are tough, stringy, fibrous bands of scar tissue that connect two pieces of body tissue not normally attached to each other. They may interfere with the normal motion of the intestine, and may cause blockages and obstructions. Not all patients form adhesions, but when they occur, they can cause abdominal pain, vomiting, and constipation.

Besides blockages caused by adhesions, blockages can also result from certain foods or from muscle spasms. You need to consult with your doctor to determine the difference between blockages caused by adhesions and other sorts of blockages. In particular, if you have an ostomy, working closely with a doctor who is experienced in treating ostomies is crucial.

Jan Gray found herself facing this dilemma after surgery. Here she relates her experience:

Jan's Story

A month after my first bowel resection, at age fifty-seven, I developed a blockage. The pain and discomfort were profound. The physician mercifully directed me to the hospital immediately upon learning of my pain. The intestinal blockage was more painful than any part of the cancer incident. (It was more painful than being in labor!)

I was told that blockages are not uncommon. The physician suggested two options once my pain was medicated: to reopen the surgical incision, or, if possible, to manage the pain and hope that the blockage was a "kink" in the intestine and that with time it would "unkink." I remember thinking of my intestines as a garden hose that had a kink. I asked the doc about perhaps using Velcro when closing the incision in case he needed to open it again. (Rats! Not possible.)

I was game to try sitting out the blockage, if possible. Of course, nothing I ate could go down. The saying "what goes up must come down" was reversed: What went down came up. On my fifth day in the hospital, the doc recommended we do a surgical procedure the next day to relieve the blockage. I was both relieved to think the end was in sight and apprehensive about undergoing a second surgery so soon after the first. I was more relieved on day six when it started to become evident that an "unkinking" was happening! Day seven revealed a total unblocking of the intestine. I so appreciated my doctor's patience and willingness to encourage me day after day to stay the course. The hospital staff managed the pain and discomfort; the doc recognized my ability to endure, and the outcome was wonderful!

In the back of my mind, although the medical staff thought there was no substantive information supporting this theory, I believed the blockage developed when I returned home from surgery. I began eating "like normal," as I had been advised to do. In my case, "normal" included fresh, raw veggies and fruits and whole grains. Following the blockage, I sought advice from a nutritionist well-versed in whole foods. For the first few weeks I prepared and ate steamed vegetables, fruits, and easily digested grains. I also ate baby foods and toddler foods during the first week. I progressively added back the normal parts of my diet over a few more weeks: grains, meats, raw foods.

Shortly before my second colon-cancer surgery I was invited to take part in a study about avoiding a blockage. I signed up immediately and participated with great enthusiasm, hoping I was getting the test element and not the placebo. I am unaware of the results of the study. I hope it was a huge success and that patients can now avoid an intestinal blockage.

Steps to Healing: Being Helped by Complementary Therapies

Some complementary therapies can be used alongside conventional healing therapies as a recommended part of your health plan. However, if you are experiencing nausea, pain, or anxiety following your surgery, you need to call your doctor. Complementary therapies may offer great benefits, but it is important to be at least somewhat sceptical before buying into a product or method that is not under any form of government regulation.

Acupuncture is one of the most common forms of complementary medicine. During acupuncture, needles are placed into strategic points of the body to relieve pain and other negative side effects you might be feeling. Proponents of acupuncture believe that disease results from an imbalance in the body of *qi* (sometimes spelled *chi*, and pronounced "chee"), the energy present in all living things. The safest way to approach acupuncture is to make sure the acupuncturist and your doctor are working together. You should also verify the credentials of your acupuncturist with the state health department. Check with your insurance company to find out if acupuncture is covered in your health plan.

Besides acupuncture, several other therapies purport to heal the body through the manipulation of energy. Such treatments are collectively referred to as *energy work,* and two of these are *reiki* and *qi gong* (pronounced "chee kung"). Julie Weaver says:

> I absolutely attribute my additional healing to reiki, which involves channeling the energy that surrounds us into whoever may need an additional healing boost. Anyone can learn how to use reiki. I did reiki on an open wound that resulted from a hospital infection. I was at home, and the home-health-care nurses visited daily for five weeks to treat the wound. The wound healed "textbook perfectly," as one of the nurses said, and she attributed it to the reiki therapy. The scar is minimal and flexible. My surgeon said, "This healed as if I had never taken out the staples."

Julie also went to a qi gong practitioner. She is convinced the sessions helped her to maintain energy after chemo.

Supplements and/or herbal remedies that promise to revitalize and strengthen your immune system should be looked upon with suspicion. The anticancer effects of megavitamins, shark cartilage, essiac, and coffee enemas so far remain unproven. More dangerously, some herbs or supplements can interact negatively with some medications. It is a good practice to check with your doctor before introducing a new substance into your body. Some substances that are currently being studied for their preventive properties against cancer include estrogen, folic acid, and selenium.

Many forms of complementary healing can offer relaxation and relief from anxiety. *Aromatherapy, massage, spiritual healing, hypnotherapy, and biofeedback* may help you to regulate negative aftereffects of surgery by changing the way you feel. As discussed in Chapter 5, *visualization techniques* can be effective for managing anxiety and promoting a healing sense of relaxation and peace. Ruth, who we heard from in the last chapter, recalls an experience that occurred while she was working with visualization:

> On one particular occasion I visualized that I suddenly went to a very rocky, very windy shore. I could see huge, threatening waves surrounding me. And wind. I heard lots of wind. I stepped out onto the water, and I can remember hearing myself howling with fear, but my determination to get to the opposite shore overcame my fear. I felt panic, and I was crying hysterically, but I continued to walk, right across the water, to where I could see a sunny beach of smooth, warm, white sand with a grove of tall pine trees in the background. When I finally made it to the other side, I curled up on the warm sand and went to sleep. I interpreted the experience as the other shore representing life, since I worked so hard to get there. I continue to remember my vision as a promise of life.

§ § §

Jane Nielsen, who we met in Chapters 1 and 3, offers the following advice on becoming part of the healing solution:

> Since my cancer diagnosis, I have become more aware of the contributions I can make toward my own health and well-being. Like most people on a quest for healing, I question what is in my control and what is not. As a cancer survivor, the questions come at such a rapid pace it is clearly overwhelming. I found it helpful, therefore, to simply concentrate on the ways I can help my body restore and maintain its natural functioning, peace, and serenity. These include:
>
> ♦ finding a sacred space to meditate and making it a daily practice to do so

- ◆ honoring my body as a sacred vessel, carefully considering what I put into it (I now eat a higher percentage of whole and organic foods)

- ◆ intentionally bolstering my immune system with cancer-fighting antioxidants, via food and supplements

- ◆ exercising regularly to promote circulation of blood and lymph, which carry essential fuels to my cells and eliminate waste

- ◆ drinking more water to allow my body's natural processes and defenses to work at an optimal level

- ◆ improving my sleep by increasing my serotonin levels. Since my exposure to sunshine is limited, I use broad-spectrum lightbulbs to stimulate my own serotonin production.

- ◆ surrounding myself with positive friends, healthy plants (yes, they have names), and selfless activities that reinforce my sense of self-worth. I've correspondingly removed the negative, unhealthy influences from my life that drained my energy.

- ◆ deepening spiritually. My faith and my faith community reinforce my belief that I am not alone, but rather am connected to a Higher Power, a loftier purpose. My experience with cancer has given me the clarity to really appreciate the gifts that I feel called on to use to be a part of the solution, not part of the problem.

¶ ¶ ¶

Good healing can come from adequate nutrition, rest, relaxation, and avoiding stress. So far, however, none of those factors have been proven to "cure" cancer, only to lead to a better recovery.

Alternative methods of healing can certainly be effective and soothing, but it's also important to bear in mind the Latin warning *caveat emptor* ("buyer beware"). No doubt there is a strong mind-body connection in healing. Acupuncture and biofeedback are proven methods of relieving pain. However, just because they're labeled "alternative" or "natural" does not mean they are harmless. I once went to an acupuncturist who caused me a great deal of pain while trying to increase the energy flow in my colon. Even though I informed her of my ileostomy, she did not get the concept that my small intestine was not hooked up to my colon.

"Cures" that are improperly researched may at best end up costing you money and, at the worst, cause you unnecessary harm. Review the section "Questionable Treatments" in Chapter 5 for strategies to help you distinguish the "snake oil" from legitimate products or methods.

Positive Options after Surgery

◆ Follow all postoperative directions. Call your doctor if you have any questions.

◆ Your body has been through a lot. Give yourself plenty of time to rest and recuperate. Enjoy the good times whenever you can.

◆ Discard any unused medicines left over from your hospital stay. Always read the labels carefully before taking any pills.

◆ Alternative methods of healing can be beneficial, but check the credentials of anyone administering therapy as well as the costs of any treatment. Make sure there is two-way communication between your complementary-therapy practitioner and your doctors.

◆ Join a support group. Turn to supportive friends and family. If there is no colorectal cancer support group in your area, contact ACE (see Resources).

Chapter 8

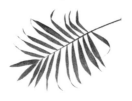

The Challenges of Chemotherapy

Cancer survivors know that life is a delicate balance between preservation and destruction. The beauty and power of our souls have been matched against the blight of cancer and the distress of treatment. A reassuring voice, a human touch, and the knowledge that other people were watching over us were by far the most powerful antidotes against the destruction of our spirit. This was a time in our lives when we most fully realized how much the help of other people could keep us from sinking. This was especially true for those of us who were required to return to chemotherapy following surgery.

Returning to Chemotherapy

I was scheduled to resume chemotherapy in earnest after my daughter Laura's wedding. Since I had been diagnosed with stage III cancer, current protocols dictated that adjuvant chemotherapy be given after surgery to destroy any remaining errant cancer cells. By this time, I was becoming familiar with the maze of Medicine Land. I knew my way around and was more skilled at expressing my needs effectively. I was taking a proactive role in my health care and learning to use the same vocabulary as my doctors and nurses. That improved our communication.

Totally unexpected was the fact that my most supportive group in regards to my health were my doctors, my nurses, and other patients. I was welcomed back to chemotherapy like a traveler returning home. Going in for treatments was usually an upbeat and positive experience. "How was the wedding?" Dr. Sborov, my oncologist, asked me. The nurses asked, "Did you bring any pictures?"

When I entered the room to get my dose of chemo, several sea-green Naugahyde lounging chairs arranged in a circle were occupied by other people like me, coming in for prescribed dosages of whatever type of chemo they needed. The atmosphere wasn't depressing. The conversations were frequently chatty; we talked about the latest book or the hottest movie. There was joking and catching up on the news of the week. Unbelievably, there were few complaints about the needles attached to our veins. Some people whose chemo required that they be there for hours watched videos, while others slept. The nurses and I swapped stories that made us laugh. Nobody dwelt on the negative or went overboard with too much sympathy. When I finished a series of blood tests and was walking out with three bandages on my arm, Dr. Sborov came by and remarked, "Looks like you got in a fight with a cat."

Traveling the Chemotherapy Highway

Nobody can tell you what going through chemotherapy will be like for you. In this chapter I've recorded my own experience, which might shed some light by telling you what I found helpful. Later in the chapter, Dan's story presents another perspective on the struggle. In both our cases, family and friends sustained us. There were times when each of us was tempted to give up and quit the work of chemotherapy. At such moments, it is imperative that we as cancer patients get support and cheerleading from medical staff and other people, and draw deep on our own resources to keep going.

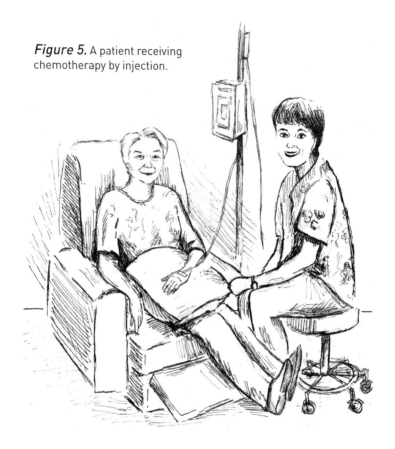

Figure 5. A patient receiving chemotherapy by injection.

At first, going through chemotherapy seemed like a gondola ride. I would go in for my treatments, knowing that competent people were steering the boat. If I had a day or two when I felt slightly under the weather, I would just lie back and enjoy the scenery. The majority of the week I felt almost like my old self. On those days, I would play some golf with the assistance of a cart or meet friends for lunch or dinner.

I didn't fully realize until I had cancer how easy my life had been. I was blessed with good health and abundant energy. I was used to a luxurious stream of comfort. I never knew how quickly the current could change. People go through chemotherapy with varying levels of difficulty. Having an ileostomy complicated my responses to treatments, but, as I found out later, some of the problems I encountered could have been avoided.

By the middle of August, it seemed as if my gondola was being sandbagged by unexpected cargo, making it harder for me to keep my balance. I could no longer just be a passive passenger; I needed to make adjustments to keep my equilibrium. This required problem solving. Even though an oncologist will monitor your blood levels, observe your stamina, and be on the lookout for any severe depression or tiredness, you need to do your part if you want to weather the storm with the least damage.

For me, it was a wise decision not to have my ileostomy reversed until after the chemotherapy was over. I was having daily bouts with diarrhea but was only aware of it because of slight cramping and the contents of my bag. I felt like I had a constant case of the flu. I became progressively dehydrated. I was told to keep drinking water, but that was hard to do once I was nauseated. My white blood cell count dropped, signaling a decline in the function of my immune system, but also signaling that the chemo was doing its job. I was given two hours of intravenous fluids and skipped that week of chemotherapy. A few days later, I lay in bed for hours over several days in a row, just trying to be still so I could get some relief from the cramps caused by diarrhea. I had always thought of myself as a person who had a zest for life. There I was, listless, enduring pain and not knowing what to do.

I decided to call Dr. Sborov. He gave me a prescription for an antidiarrheal drug. Like magic, the pain disappeared. I hadn't realized that even though I had an ileostomy, I could get help for the discomfort of diarrhea. From that point on, I took the antidiarrheal drug regularly, which helped me immensely. My first real problem had been solved, and I was strongly back on course.

Nausea was my next, most immediate, problem. At the end of August, when I reached my first two-week break in the six-week chemo regimen, I almost cancelled. Once again, I called the doctor's office, and this time I got a prescription for antinausea pills. I was immensely grateful for feeling better. I came back from my vacation from chemo treatments strengthened by rest and determined that my second cycle of chemo would go even more smoothly than the first. So far, so good.

Things That Help

You might hear your oncologist refer to your *neutrophils* as a measure of how well you are keeping up your immunities. Neutrophils are specialized white blood cells that fight infection. Problematic blood cell counts are not unexpected. It only means that the chemo is working, at least on healthy cells. (Hopefully, if there are any residual bad ones, the chemo is taking care of those too.)

It's helpful to track your progress just like your oncologist is doing, even to the point of keeping a journal to identify predictable patterns. You will find that even this abnormal life has a rhythm to it. Resting for a day or two after each treatment helps restore your reserves of energy. When you have good days, do the things you most enjoy doing. It might take an effort on your part to partake in pleasurable activities, but they are distracting and will help to raise your morale. As much as possible, surround yourself with people who give you the most energy and lift up your spirits.

Mouth sores are a common side effect of chemotherapy. Most people never think of calling their dentist for help while undergoing chemo, but a dentist can order prescriptive medications that can ease the pain. Call a cancer center or do some research on the Internet for suggestions about how to combat mouth sores. A non-alcoholic toothpaste and a child's toothbrush can help if the regular kinds become too irritating for you to use. Ice chips are a wonderful way to keep your mouth moist. Sugarless Popsicles can become a therapeutic treat. If possible, keep flossing.

At some point during treatment, it's not unusual for patients to find they are struggling with a distaste for food and increased tiredness. You may find that your desire for sex, just like your appetite for food, diminishes temporarily. Be sure to tell your partner that your need for tenderness and love hasn't changed, however.

Oddly enough, even while going through chemotherapy, I could still laugh and feel happy, and all of my ACE colleagues report the same thing. The kindness and love shown by other people can make up for a lot of things that may seem lacking in your life right now. Phone calls, letters, and cards can be day brighteners. You may find yourself experiencing plenty of Hallmark moments that would make good commercials. Prayer and listening to inspirational tapes while resting can give solace.

I managed well until the middle of my second cycle, and then my whole body bogged down. The antidiarrheal drugs were no longer doing their job. Going downstairs to start a load of wash was a major undertaking. I couldn't seem to keep food in my system for long, and I lost my appetite entirely. Even water was repugnant. I rarely got sick, but I was nauseated most of the time. Hamburger was like rubber and bread tasted like sawdust. Getting adequate nutrition was becoming a problem, and I didn't even realize it. My throat was dry most of the time. Well-meaning people kept pushing food in front of me, but that just seemed to make it worse. I was having progressively more difficulty swallowing, so I resorted to eating only ice cream and yogurt malts. Anything chocolate and creamy was appealing to me. Fortified, prepared liquid food (like Ensure) would have helped my nutritional needs, but I gagged when I tried to get it down.

Maybe because of the stress, I was confused at times. I found it hard to concentrate. People who have been there call it "chemobrain." I've never read any research on the phenomenon, but I experienced it. I began feeling separated from people, like I had been invaded by body snatchers. My husband and my children took over all of the household duties. Every day was a struggle to overcome depression, but sometimes it was a relief just to go with the sorrow. If I stayed too long with my negative thoughts, however, they seemed to weigh me down further. More and more I felt as if I were sinking, headed for a whirlpool I wanted to avoid.

It was just a matter of time until the diarrhea and my lack of a proper diet caused my body to rebel. I spent one morning at the hospital with a partial blockage in my intestine. The food I was forcing myself to eat was not digesting as it should. Vicki, one of the enterostomal nurses, irrigated my ileostomy by introducing running water into the bowel to help expel the waste material. That opened me up, but it was necessary for me to go on a liquid diet for the next day.

I started to lose my will to complete chemotherapy. It was my daughter Jennifer who came through with a solution.

My husband, Dave, and I had taken Jennifer to dinner. When the food arrived, I had such revulsion to it I told them I was ready to give up taking any more treatments. My daughter listened very carefully to what I was saying and remarked, "You know, Mom, your symptoms sound just like those of some of the athletes I have coached: dry mouth, inability to swallow, and nausea. Those are all signs of dehydration. Could that be your problem?"

"No," I said with certainty. "I drink at least eight glasses of water a day."

Dave corrected me, "You know, you really don't."

I tried to protest, but he came back with, "You *pour* yourself eight glasses a day, but I've been watching you, and you only drink a little of each glass before you pour it down the sink."

I realized, at that moment, that what he was saying was true.

Jenny added, "Dehydration can make you nauseous and very sick, Mom. It's serious."

That made sense to me. I was probably dehydrated. The diarrhea from chemotherapy can cause dehydration, and I remembered reading that a person with an ileostomy was even more susceptible. Acting on this assumption, I drank a cup of cocoa and several glasses of water throughout the night. By the next morning, I experienced a transformation. I was no longer as nauseous. I began to eat some real food.

I finished the last two treatments doing much better. I still kept taking antidiarrheal drugs, and I was also drinking (not just pouring!) at least eight glasses of water a day. My appetite was poor, but at least I could make myself ingest food better than before. However, I was still having trouble swallowing. I was drinking soups or hot fudge yogurt malts, and I began putting a protein powder in them. I managed to gain a few pounds, and Dr. Sborov was pleased by my progress. Gradually, I began to regain my optimism; I went from feeling fearful to being a little euphoric. I realized I had turned the corner and just had a little bit more distance to go before I would be on safe shores once again. This is when I started earnestly to improve my nutrition, get more exercise, and take regular naps every day. Gradually I became stronger in body as well as in spirit.

But I didn't do it alone. It was sometimes hard for me to accept help from other people, but that's what I did. Dave drove me to the rest of my treatments. My oldest daughter, Tami, rallied Laura and Jennifer to take turns cleaning our house. My brother Red suggested I use the time to write a biography of my mom. My sister and friends wrote me wonderful letters. Some of my friends apologized for sharing their problems with me, but the truth was that I needed to think about other things, not just my struggle with cancer. It was important for me to feel a part of life and to be able to help others as much as I could.

I learned two important lessons from the experience: There are many things a patient can do to minimize the devastating side effects of chemotherapy, and there is nothing quite so restorative as the help of others when life gets scary and overwhelming.

Other members of our group have stories of overcoming harsh side effects and learning what to do to counteract them. Ruth Edstrom was one of the few people I talked to who did lose her hair, probably due to the potency of the three drugs she was taking. When it finally started to come out in clumps, she decided to shave it all off, rather than watch it thin out bit by bit. She recalls watching *It's a Wonderful Life* and other uplifting movies as a way to keep her spirits up. Many of us found relief by going to support groups or getting massages. For many people, a healing touch can help them feel more energized.

Dan's Story

You met Dan in Chapter 2. He was twenty-five when he was diagnosed with stage IV colorectal cancer. That was more than seven years ago, but he still has a vivid memory of the challenges he faced with chemotherapy. As he recalls:

> After being diagnosed I was in the hospital for seventeen days because of a staph infection, which added about two months to my healing process. I actually lost my hearing in one ear because I was so frail that some part of my inner ear shrank and caused a temporary hearing loss. That was strange.
>
> I remember when I could begin to take showers by myself. I was staying at my parents' house because I could not pack the incision or get around very well on my own. One morning I was in the shower and my dad was standing outside keeping an eye on me. I passed out and fell through the glass door to the floor. Remarkably, the door did not break but just slammed open against the wall as I fell into it. We are still amazed when we think about the incident. From that day forward, I started noticing that maybe someone was keeping an eye on me. I am not religious, but I do believe in some sort of higher power or energy. I really believe it was my Grandpa Joe watching over me. He died of the same form of cancer that I was diagnosed with. He and I have always had a unique connection through our similarities. He could play any instrument he picked up and was very talented. I am the same way. I play guitar and piano and have never taken a lesson. It just comes naturally to me. I think of him often.

All of these negative experiences caused Dan to take a different direction in the months to come. He decided that he could feel sorry and angry about his situation, or he could face it head on and be as positive as possible. "Don't get me wrong," he admits. "I had plenty of angry and sad days, but overall I always came back to my decision to try a little harder to have a good attitude."

Dan's chemotherapy began two months later than originally planned. As he remembers:

I was very nervous. Because my cancer was so advanced, I feared that I would just get sicker before I died. For a few days, I actually contemplated just living out my life and trying to get in a few good months before it was over. I have never shared with anyone how close I was to that decision. But, after many hours of thinking, I decided I had too much to live for and there was no way this could be my time to leave. Actually, my niece and nephew had the most impact on me in making that decision. I just couldn't imagine that someday they would understand that I just gave up. I am very much a role model to them. What kind of message would my giving up have sent?

Because I was so young, my doctors were very confident that I could find the attitude, strength, and courage to beat this, even if it came back. I could probably sustain more surgeries and treatments. Their confidence helped me to see the light at the end of the tunnel. I figured, after all I had been through over the preceding two months, that nothing could be worse. It could only get better—from a pain-in-the-butt perspective, that is. I also had family around me who never stopped moving forward with a positive attitude. They protected me from hearing about the deaths of other cancer patients I knew. They pushed me when I wanted to stop. They left me alone when I needed to be alone. They drove me to every treatment. They watched me deteriorate but understood that my doing so was necessary to kill the cancer. I was very fortunate to have such a strong circle around me, in particular my dad, Ben. I still don't understand how he sat and watched his son go through what I did and never showed any anger or a negative attitude. What an incredible man.

Dan's chemotherapy lasted seven or eight months because he had to stop a couple of times between cycles. When certain blood count levels get too high or too low, doctors may delay a patient's treatments simply because the patient is too sick or weak for it to be safe. Since Dan was diagnosed with a stage IV cancer, he was given the highest dosages of the strongest medicines he could sustain in order to save his life. Incredibly, he survived. Through it all, Dan tried to be as positive as he could about his ordeals.

I was lucky—I did not totally lose my hair. There were good days and bad days. My chemo regimen consisted of a one week on, then two weeks off. The week following the treatments I would begin to get sick, and the second week it would get worse. Then when the third week came around, I would start feeling better and BAM!, it was time to get zapped again. I remember getting awful sores in my mouth; they made it impossible to eat or swallow. Nausea came and went although I did not actually get sick much. It just always felt like I was about to. Then came the other drugs: one to help anxiety, one to help with nausea, another to help with the sores, another to help me sleep. Some worked, some didn't. With regard to combating side effects, I encourage people to keep trying, because sometimes it took my trying different drugs before I found one that actually worked for me.

Dan did not use any alternative methods for healing. He says:

A few people who had the vitamin/supplement answer to my woes approached me. My oncologist told me that I could pretty much take a multivitamin everyday and it would have the same effect as taking forty-five supplements. You just end up peeing all of the extra substances (and the money) right out of your body. I did use some meditation exercises to help me relax. I would light some candles and sit or lie down in a very comfortable chair or couch. Then I would breathe deeply and imagine that I was blowing the cancer out of my body. I would actually visualize it leaving my body through my nose and mouth. This helped me a lot. When I felt nausea or anxiety I would do this, and it really seemed to take away some of the symptoms. I also listened to rainforest music, which helped me relax.

❡ ❡ ❡

Most cancer survivors I've spoken with say that when chemotherapy and radiation treatments ended, they experienced tremendous joy and relief. But that doesn't mean our lives instantly returned to normal. For one thing, we lived with the effects of our treatments for quite some time. Other new challenges emerged as well, some of which are covered in the next two chapters.

Like a soldier returning from war, it may take you a while to realize you are out of danger once you complete cancer treatment. Give yourself time to adjust and to recover from some of the harsher aftereffects.

Positive Options for Going Through Chemotherapy

◆ Focus on the present. Let go of minor problems. Live as well as you can.

◆ Be kind to yourself. Let the kindness of others help to buoy you up.

◆ Enhance your life with peace, faith, spirituality, meditation, deep breathing, and imagery.

◆ Express your emotions. Cultivate thoughts that encourage you to heal. Accept that you will have some negative or down times too.

◆ Clearly communicate your symptoms to your oncologist. Do not assume that just because you are going through chemotherapy you have to be sick. Effective medicine is available to help with side effects.

◆ Track your progress in a journal. Not only is doing so therapeutic, but you may also be able to identify helpful, predictable patterns.

◆ Do as much as you can to preserve your health. A dentist knowledgeable about cancer can give you help for preventative measures against mouth sores.

◆ Make sure you are getting adequate nutrition in your diet. Consider consulting with a dietician or nutritionist who has worked with chemotherapy patients.

- Dehydration can become a problem. Take seriously the suggestion that you should drink at least eight glasses of water a day.

- Don't forget to
  - rest, especially right after each treatment
  - relax, by doing the things you most enjoy
  - reach out and stay involved with other people; accept and appreciate their help.

- Remember that someday you can pass on what you have learned to someone else.

Chapter 9

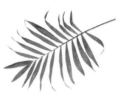

Possible Complications
after Treatment

It has almost become a cultural cliché that those of us who have cancer are supposed to behave like gladiators and "put up a good fight" against this disease. We are, of course, up against a rampage of cancer cells within our body, rather than an external enemy, but aren't we also facing questions of life and death?

It's important to remember that no matter how courageously we fight, we may not, in the end, be given a "thumbs up." Complications can develop over which we have no control, and predictions of there being no recurrence are sometimes inexplicably overturned. The most valiant heroes aren't always successful in overcoming cancer and should not be made to feel they are to blame if, despite their efforts, they are given a "thumbs down" and cancer takes over their body. The reality of this journey is that we are all struggling to find our way while at the same time trying to live the best life we can.

The word *fight* is appropriate only in the sense of rallying determination, resisting the loss of hope, making ourselves strong, learning all we can about what we have to face, and adapting the mental attitude of victor rather than victim. Staying stuck in anger will not destroy the cancer cells within us. Establishing a peaceful state of mind, however, will make our struggles easier to bear and give our immune systems every chance to restore our health.

After surgery has made divots in our intestines, and as our treatments are being completed, those of us who have survived find ourselves facing new challenges while we try to regain our balance. When a person gets to this point, "winning" means making the most of life, no matter what the long-term outcome. Winning becomes a quest to make every day count. That is the victory.

Cancer is a wretched disease, but it has no power over the human spirit.

Ileostomies and Colostomies

Let's review some terminology. As discussed in Chapter 6, an *ostomy* is an artificial opening in the body that creates a new pathway for the body to discard waste. The type of ostomy you receive will depend on the location of the operation. For colorectal cancer, there are two main types of ostomies that can be created during surgery: an *ileostomy* or a *colostomy* (see Figure 6, on the facing page). Either one can be permanent or temporary.

Typically, a colostomy is positioned to the left of the navel, and an ileostomy is positioned to the right. The consistency and frequency of discharge will depend on the location of the ostomy. Waste materials are collected in a bag that is stuck onto the skin with an adhesive. A skin barrier is used to protect the stoma and the area around it. (The *stoma* is the part of the intestine that is brought to the surface of the abdomen to make the new opening.)

An ileostomy, which is what I have, is connected to the ileum (the lowest portion of the small intestine). With an ileostomy, partially digested food that has passed through the stomach and small intestine is diverted via the stoma into a small plastic bag. The waste materials are more liquid than they would be with a colostomy, and they are highly acidic, which kills off most of the bacteria.

One of the problems with an ileostomy or a colostomy is that the digestion of food is continuous. Sometimes, after a meal, the

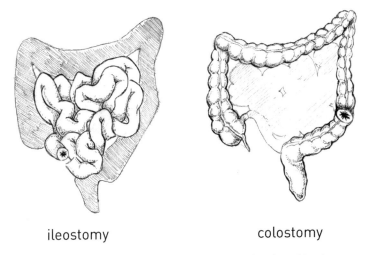

ileostomy   colostomy

Figure 6. A colostomy is usually created in the sigmoid colon (right); an ileostomy is created from the small bowel (left).

food may come happily gurgling out of your intestine, making sounds similar to those of a stomach growling. You can help to keep the sounds of this process under control by avoiding gas-producing foods and (when out in public) taking a mild gas suppressant before meals.

Most people who need an ostomy after colorectal cancer surgery have a colostomy. A colostomy is created by surgery when part of the colon has been removed and resected. It can be located at any point where the surgery took place. Just as in an ileostomy, waste products will pass through the stoma into a bag, but the consistency and odor of the waste will be more like feces. Some people who have colostomies located within the lower, sigmoid colon prefer to irrigate the bowel (introducing water into the bowel through the ostomy in order to clean out any waste material) instead of using a bag.

Brenda Elsagher, who has a permanent colostomy from having colorectal cancer, prefers the process of irrigating. "The advantage of irrigating was training the colon to be active only during the procedure," she says. "This meant I could return to work and not worry about stool in my pouch. Odors were no longer a problem because my new pouch had a charcoal filter and sound muffler built into it. When gas was expelled, no one else had to know about it."

Brenda imbues the irrigation process with her ready sense of making everything as fun as it can be. As she describes it, "I began making my bathroom a sacred place where I could escape my small children for a short period. I decided to make it quality time." Brenda had her husband, Bahgat, hang a shelf where she keeps stationery, magazines, writing material, and makeup to use during her "irrigation hour."

Brenda quips, "It's not so bad having a colostomy. I just can't find shoes to match my bag."

Ostomates (people who have ostomies) have a wide variety of appliances from which to choose. You may prefer bags you can dispose of every three or four days. You should empty the bag every time it is one-third full. It is a good practice to carry a small plastic bottle, fill it with about a quarter cup of water (not hot water!), and rinse the bag every time you empty it during a regular "bathroom break." Using deodorizing drops makes this process odorless. It takes less than half a minute to complete the whole process. That's it. You may be rather clumsy doing this operation at first; it's easy to forget that when the bag isn't sealed, the material in it can pour out. (The stool in an ileostomy is more liquid.)

With an ostomy, you can go anywhere, swim, soak in a hot tub, ski, and work at any task that does not require lifting more than twenty pounds. If you have trouble finding clothes that fit your new figure, consult a personal shopper at a department store to get some ideas.

Some people are afraid to travel with an ostomy. A book titled *Yes We Can!* (see Resources) is full of good tips for travelers. It directs you to resources around the world where you can find colorectal surgeons and enterostomal nurses. There are ostomy appliance suppliers in almost every country. Flying is no problem, but all ostomates who travel must bear in mind one explicit caution: Keep your supplies with you at all times. Occasionally airlines misplace baggage. Your ostomy supplies need to travel in your carry-on bag rather than in your checked luggage. *Yes We Can!* also includes an explanation of ostomies in different languages, in case you need to explain your situation to security officers in a foreign land.

Blockages

People who have ileostomies in particular have to watch their diet, chew their food carefully, and still make sure they eat a balanced diet. Blockages can occur when the ileostomy fails to function for short periods of time. If you are having cramps and are vomiting, you need to get immediate care by medical personnel. However, there are some measures you can take to treat an obstruction before it progresses to that point: Sometimes a warm bath, drinking a glass of pure grape juice, or massaging your abdomen will be enough to relax your intestine and let the food pass through. You can also try removing your pouch and cutting a larger hole in the bag to accommodate a swollen stoma. If that doesn't work, you can try to irrigate your stoma at home.

Vicki, one of my enterostomal nurses, taught me how to clear a blockage by irrigating the opening of my small intestine with water. I remember my reaction to the whole experience; to be honest, the whole process of irrigation was frightening. Vicki placed a slender, lubricated rubber tube in my hand, sixteen-inches long, red-orange in color, and a quarter-inch in diameter. "Are you sure I'm not going to damage myself when I do this?" I asked. "You'll be just fine," she said with assurance, "There is nothing here that will hurt you."

Under her guidance I attached a plastic pump full of water to one end of the tube and then fed the other end of the tube into my belly through my stoma. It snaked its way down into a space I never before knew existed.

"Think of yourself as a professional mechanic flushing and then siphoning the sludge out of the carburetor of a car," she suggested. "That's no good," I said. "I'm terrible at fixing machines, and that goes double for trying to make repairs on my own body." "You'll be fine," Vicki repeated. "It doesn't hurt, does it?" "No," I had to admit. It just looked bad.

The Be-Attitudes of Having an Ostomy

Normally functioning ostomies can give you freedom from the agonies of a diseased bowel. They can offer you complete control over your life. No one would ever claim that adjusting to living with an ostomy is easy, but those of us who have learned to live with one would be the first to acknowledge the blessings of doing so. I call the lessons I have learned the "be-attitudes" of having an ostomy. They are as follows:

Be educated. It takes time to find out that you can still have an excellent life with an ostomy. Knowledge will empower you.

Be prepared. Your motto should be, "Ostomy supplies: Don't leave home without them!" Carry an extra pouch with adhesive at all times. If you go on a trip, double the supplies you think you will need, and carry them with you rather than packing them in checked baggage. Have the phone number of an ostomy supplier wherever you go. Do your ordering on a regular basis.

Be on guard. Watch your diet, especially if you have an ileostomy. In that case, select and chew your food carefully. Avoid strenuous lifting. Wear a belt for protection when engaged in contact sports.

Be up on all the new equipment. Ostomy appliance manufacturers consistently improve their products. Do you have a particular problem with your ostomy? Call the manufacturer or contact your enterostomal nurse.

Be nice to yourself. Give yourself credit for doing as well as you can while adjusting to an ostomy. Social anxiety, performance anxiety during sex, and excessive worrying can be self-fulfilling prophecies. Tune in to your emotional state. The more you are aware of negative feelings, the more you have an opportunity to alter them.

Be patient with others who do not understand. How long did it take you to learn about ostomies? You have a golden opportunity to help others become educated. People will generally ask only what you are willing to share, but if you feel a question is too intrusive, you can tell them it is a matter you don't want to discuss at that moment.

Become an advocate! Overcoming the difficulties of living with an ostomy is an ongoing process. Share what you learn with others—join a local chapter of the United Ostomy Association.

When a Temporary Ostomy Becomes Permanent

As I neared the end of my chemotherapy treatments about seven months after my surgery, I had an appointment with my colorectal surgeon to discuss the reversal of my ileostomy. Instead of being happy at this prospect, I actually dreaded it. Radiation proctitis had weakened the lining of my rectum and augmented the pain of any intrusive test I had to undergo. Heavy bleeding after any rectal exam had become a regular occurrence and had become progressively more painful.

Two days before one of my final appointments, Dr. Nemer's receptionist called me to come in for a special consultation. This was an unusual summons. I fearfully pondered what the surgeon might want to tell me. When I entered his office, I could see his expression was grim.

"I'm sorry," he began, "but I'm having problems advocating reversing your ileostomy. Only 5 percent of patients have severe chronic proctitis," he continued, "and you are one of them."

I didn't want to hear what I was hearing. A silent voice within me protested. "Would it help to wait?" I asked feebly.

He measured his words so there would be no misunderstanding. "No. The damage to what's left of your rectum is irreversible.

It probably won't be getting much better than it is now."

For almost a minute, I couldn't speak. He finally said, "You might want to consider keeping the ileostomy permanent, unless you are willing to go through much suffering to try to do without it. Even in the most ideal situation, after having most of your rectum removed, you would be battling some diarrhea and incontinence. Now, with the continuing proctitis, those problems would only make the transition much harder to bear."

"One thing I have to know. Will having an ostomy shorten my life expectancy?"

He didn't hesitate. "Not a day. Not even a day."

I was choking on my words, but I had to ask one more question. "What would you do?"

"I'm a doctor. I have to be in control of my life. I would stay with the ileostomy."

Although I desperately wanted to avoid having a permanent ileostomy, I understood the wisdom of what he was saying. I thought back to all the pain I suffered every time I had a test involving my rectum. On a regular basis I suffered a lot of discomfort if I stood on my feet for too long. The thought of enduring diarrhea or incontinence on top of what I was already experiencing was grim. I told him I needed to think about it. We made plans to meet again in a week.

For the next few days I stayed at home, feeling depressed. I actually wondered if life was worth all of this suffering. I was angry. At whom, for what, I wasn't sure. Was I mad at all the radiation I had been given? That was a question I repeatedly asked myself. But wasn't I cancer free six months after my first diagnosis? So maybe the radiation had been necessary.

Still, I couldn't get beyond the grief I was feeling from knowing that my body would be altered forever.

Not knowing where to turn, I made an appointment to see Vicki and Julie. They didn't give me any advice, but just listened as I vented my anguish. Then they offered another perspective I had not considered. "You know, Carol, most of the people we see here are grateful for an ostomy. Their lives have been miserable with colitis or other colorectal diseases. An ostomy enables them to have a beautiful life. It sounds like that might be the case for you, as well."

What they were saying made a lot of sense. "Think about it," they said. "On a daily basis, has the ostomy been so hard to live with?"

I played a rerun of the last six months in my memory. Except for the problems caused by the blockages, which were mostly caused by dehydration, I had been saved from all the pain I probably would have encountered from diarrhea. "I guess I have to admit that, 98 percent of the time, the ostomy has not been a problem," I said. "I suppose the thought of having it forever is what's making it so hard."

They understood what I meant. "It's probably harder for you because you had different expectations, but you know, I think you've been adjusting very well to the idea."

And I had. Suddenly, it wasn't really a big deal anymore. Even though I'd thought it was going to be temporary, I was managing to do everything I wanted to do without letting it interfere with my life.

They continued to reassure me. "We can equip you with top-of-the-line appliances, and we can experiment with shapes and sizes. We will be here to give you all the help you need if you run into any more roadblocks." They added, "You might even want to consider joining a local United Ostomy Association group and going to their meetings. They're very helpful."

When I left the office, I knew I had to move on. There was no question what decision I was going to have to make. I wanted to lead the highest quality of life available to me. Some of my vanity would have to go, and my ileostomy would have to stay.

I had reached a major crossroads in my journey, and I decided to choose a path that would ensure a better way of life for me. It was crucially important that I made the decision and no one else. That fact alone gave me strength.

If there is social embarrassment accompanying a disease like colorectal cancer, there is more like a shameful silence associated with ostomies. That might be because, in the past, many ostomy appliances leaked, were cumbersome and odorous, and had to be washed and rewashed for further use. In today's world, you, as a patient, have a large number of choices among well-designed, dependable appliances, along with the option of using recyclable pouches or ones that you can discard.

Another reason why people may be afraid to talk about the fact you have an ostomy is because they are just uninformed about the topic and may believe it is a source of embarrassment to you. It's good to keep in mind that you set the stage; you may choose to keep the fact that you have an ostomy to yourself. Unless someone sees you undressed, they probably would never know. On the other hand, it makes life a lot easier to be able to talk about something you have to deal with every day of your life. The more the "secret" is out, the easier it may be for you to contend with your problems. In the process, you will have the opportunity to pass on what you have learned.

A good book about ostomies is *Positive Options for Living with Your Ostomy*, by Dr. Craig A. White (see Resources). The author, a clinical psychologist, includes a thorough discussion of how to deal with the challenging emotions that can accompany getting an ostomy.

Recurrences of Cancer

If cancer returns after thirty days from the end of the last treatment, it is called a *recurrence*. A recurrence may be indicated by slight abdominal cramps, chronic fatigue, a change in bowel habits, a distention of your stomach, spotting—the same symptoms that might have caused you to go to the doctor originally—or by some other symptom that is alarming to you. Contact your doctor if you're concerned. Sometimes recurrences are detected through routine tests, CEA levels, or examinations. There are no generalizations that can be made about recurrences, except that patients initially diagnosed with more advanced cancers are more likely to experience them. The longer you go cancer-free, the less likely you are to have a recurrence.

A recurrence may occur close to the site where your first cancer was located or farther away, in a place not initially associated with your first tumor. To treat a recurrence, your doctor may ask you to consider a second surgery. Colorectal cancer cells become immune to some chemotherapy drugs, so depending on the drugs you were treated with initially, your doctor may suggest trying new drugs. This is when you may want to participate in a clinical trial of more effective drugs than the ones you were first given.

Recurrence also brings many emotional issues with it. If you are diagnosed with a recurrence, this would be a good time to talk to a counselor knowledgeable about colorectal cancer, or to join a support group of individuals who are facing the same issue.

Jan Gray has this to say about her recurrence: "What can I control? My attitude. I could choose to take it lying down, and then I wouldn't have so far to fall. I could choose to be miserable— or to make the best of it. I could choose to listen to the negative self-doubts or decide to develop positive thoughts. The path our life will follow is never certain. We're constantly faced with curves, detours, rocky roads, and repairs. There are destinations unknown and unclear—but the support of friends and family can span the crevasses we encounter, and the journey can continue. When we are together, there is strength."

Positive Options for Dealing with Complications after Treatments

◆ Be aware that ostomies can be permanent or temporary. If you are going to have an ostomy, contact an enterostomal nurse. The United Ostomy Association (UOA) also offers resources and information that can benefit you. (For contact information, see Resources.)

- This is your body. Learn all you can about your ostomy and how to take care of it.

- Cultivate the "be-attitudes" of having an ostomy.

- Recurrences can be emotionally hard. If you are diagnosed with a recurrence, do whatever you need to do to help you through the experience.

Chapter 10

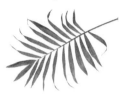

Lessons Learned from Surviving Cancer

What happens when life is supposed to become "normal" once again?

As cancer survivors, we wish we could say that once we were through with all of our treatments, and once we'd recovered from some of the harsh aftereffects, life proceeded on a steady upward path. It wasn't quite so easy. Many of us were dismayed that we didn't feel better immediately after finishing chemotherapy. The truth is that chemotherapy keeps on working for a while after you are done with treatments. Gradually, the effects wear off.

We found that new mountains needed to be scaled before we could move on to the next phase: full recovery. Most of us would say we are more appreciative of the ordinary aspects of life, some of which we used to take for granted. It's so wonderful to be able to enjoy the taste of food once again and to have renewed energy to do the things we want to do. When we gaze upon the faces we love, we immediately want to put them in the album of our minds as souvenirs of the wonderful gift of life.

There have been invaluable lessons along the way, and I want to end this book by sharing some of them.

Begin with Realistic Expectations

Give yourself time to heal. Your previous focus on trying to get well is going to change back to a focus on everyday existence. It might help to think of yourself as a vehicle that has been out of commission for some time. It makes sense to give yourself a slow, steady start. Revving yourself up too fast could stall your engine. Let yourself "idle" for a while before gunning your motor.

Occasional naps are therapeutic. Enrolling in a mild exercise program like t'ai chi or yoga contributes to a well-exercised body in addition to promoting relaxation and a positive frame of mind. Taking walks, gardening, and moderate exercise are all excellent ways to regain your strength.

Remind yourself that some tiredness is just a part of everyday living and growing older. During an ultrasound checkup with Dr. Finne, I told him, "I don't have as much stamina as I did before." "Join the club," he said, and laughed.

Many of your muscles will need gradual stretching and strengthening. Eventually, you will find the most comfortable rhythm for your lifestyle, and your endurance will slowly increase. As your health improves, your physical strength will increase— perhaps not to what it was before, but to a new "norm" for you.

Learn When to Ask for Help

The things we took for granted before—good health and being alive—are no longer "givens." Cancer was a fearsome experience, but it automatically made us part of a large group. At each medical checkpoint that comes along now, we still feel a certain amount of anxiety. But as our confidence in becoming well increases, our fears continue to lessen. In the book *Dancing in Limbo* (see Resources), the authors talk about the cruel myth that when medical treatments are completed and successful, the story ends. Feelings of uncertainty, fear, and grief, the renegotiating of relationships, and the need to revise your life are all experiences common to a survivor of cancer.

Having cancer has increased our appreciation for friends and loved ones. They were our lifelines when we needed them most, and we have a sense of gratitude for them that we will never lose. Above all, we have learned to ask friends and family for help when we need it. People don't have a crystal ball. They need to know if you want some assistance. Letting them help is a gift of your love.

There is another huge source of emotional support that may not be quite so apparent. When I was battling cancer, my calendar was dotted with appointments to see the doctors and nurses who were doing everything they could to keep me well. When it was no longer necessary for me to see them on a regular basis, I expected to feel elated. Instead, during the month following my last appointment, I found myself oddly sad. I was so thankful that the cancer seemed to be gone and that my journey with cancer was hopefully over, but I also felt scared and uneasy. I couldn't quite figure this out. I am not a dependent person, and I certainly "have a life." What was bothering me?

To gain some understanding, I enlisted the aid of an insightful psychologist at the hospital. She helped me see that the people I was leaving were the ones who guided me to safety and who were with me down the dark roads when the going was really rough. No way did I want to return to the difficulties I had before, but I would always be grateful that the doctors and nurses were there. I had been lost, and I was so glad they came along when they did. It was time for me to move on, but I know where to look if I ever need help again.

Reduce Unnecessary Stress

As a cancer survivor, you might find that your life has been changed. Confronting cancer is facing your own mortality, and once you've been there, you never forget it. We have learned to do our living in the present, to make our lives even more spontaneous and exciting than they were before.

Balancing expectations for handling the demands of stressful situations is as necessary now as it was before we were diagnosed with cancer. Being cancer survivors, however, we have overcome so many difficulties that we find we are no longer willing to tolerate negative situations that sap our enjoyment of life. In some cases this has resulted in divorce, career change, or the re-evaluation of friendships. We have learned a great deal of problem-solving skills.

We find we are constantly evaluating how we want to spend our time. We've learned the value of having a good day. Connecting with a good friend, exercising, and writing have become top priorities for me. I also have been tending to things in my environment that have bothered me for years. My husband and I hired a lawn service to plant perennial bushes and trees in our yard. They require very little work on our part and give us a beautiful view. A teenager next door cuts our lawn for us. The time to address such matters is now, not some point in the future.

This may sound contradictory, but we have also learned to slough off unsolvable problems that are really not very important. The challenge here is to know the difference. This is an area needing constant reassessment. In our ACE group, we have talked about the fact that the lack of control you sometimes feel as a patient in the course of treatment reverses itself in recovery, as you start to want to control everything. We have found that more and more we have cultivated new attitudes, making whatever changes are necessary, when possible, to improve our quality of life.

Make a Comeback from Cancer with Good Nutrition and Exercise

While there is no evidence that any food or diet can cure your cancer, eating well and exercising are crucial to your best chance for recovery. Diets high in whole grains, fruits, and vegetables are the most healthy. Fiber has benefits beyond helping to prevent colorectal cancer. Think of yourself as an athlete in training; give your body every chance to be at its best.

Maureen managed her ordeal with cancer by applying all of her athletic skills in the greatest race of her life.

Maureen's Story

Each Christmas I am reminded how lucky I am to be one year further away from the Christmas I spent at Abbott Northwestern recovering from surgery to remove the cancerous tumor in my colon. I was a twenty-eight-year-old vegetarian distance runner when I was diagnosed with stage III colon cancer on December 19, 2000.

My first symptoms appeared that fall, while I was hosting a party to watch the 2000 Olympics. I felt nauseous and vomited inexplicably. As a runner, I feel very aware of my body and how it is supposed to function. Since the symptoms continued, I kept returning to my doctor to explain that I knew something was not right. I'm so glad that I did not ignore the symptoms and that my colorectal surgeon did not dismiss my concerns but rather kept trying different tests until a colonoscopy revealed the tumor in my colon.

I feel very lucky that within one week, the problem was found, I was diagnosed, and I was in a hospital recovering. It all happened so fast I never stopped to think, "Why me?" About a month later, I was told that I could choose between two chemotherapy studies. The one I selected was scheduled to last thirty-two weeks. When I attended the mandatory prechemo class, I was in a session with a middle-aged cancer patient who was wheelchair bound and only able to move his hands to operate the mechanical chair. Here was a person who could justifiably ask, "Why me?" Many times during chemo I was reminded that I was luckier than others.

My attitude during chemo was upbeat. For me, the hardest part was the constant fatigue. I was determined to keep my life as "normal" as possible, and so I continued to work full-time as an architect. Previously, the most difficult thing I had accomplished was running a marathon. Getting through chemo was like walking a marathon—taking baby steps. As with running, there was a finish line I had my eye on: September 1, 2001. I thought all I had to do was cross that line and my life would be back to normal.

As it turned out, 2001 was the most difficult year of my life, not because of chemo but because my fifty-year-old boss, the head of the four-person architecture firm where I worked, died unexpectedly on a bike trip that spring. Paul was my mentor and a father figure to me, as my own dad had died when I was eight. His entire family had visited me in the hospital on Christmas Eve. One of the hardest parts of dealing with the tragedy was that all of my emotional energy was focused on surviving chemo, so I did not really confront my grief over his death until after I crossed the finish line in September. Unfortunately, September 11 happened one week later, which took a lot of everyone's emotional energy.

So I found that September 1st was not a line between abnormal/normal, hard/easy, or sad/happy. I no longer had a date as a goal to work toward. It was difficult to keep up the positive attitude I had embraced for nine months, but I slowly regained energy and started running again. In June 2002 I ran my third Grandma's Marathon in 3:56. I ran my fifth marathon in 2003. Paul's architecture firm was sold in 2002, and I am with another small firm now. I am engaged to be married on December 18, 2004, almost four years to the day from when I was diagnosed with cancer. Life moves forward. Whenever I watch the Olympics, I think I will feel like I have crossed another finish line.

Expect to Encounter Some Potholes of Depression

Living in Minnesota, we know about potholes. Winter ravages our highways, and even the best roads can get pitted with ruts. You can keep driving over them only so long before the constant wear and tear beats up your tires. The same is true for depression.

Since I'm a cancer survivor, the cause of many of my down moods is probably fear. I start to imagine there are insurmountable limitations in my life caused by cancer or by having an ostomy. I start to mourn what I would like to have done if this had never happened to me. Most of these feelings are in my head and limit me only because I allow them to. When I still have an occasional blockage, a cloud of negativity rains down on me for a few days. Other emotions like self-pity, martyrdom, or resentment are there too, when I least seem to want them. When I find such feelings mucking up the road, I work on not letting them accumulate, so they won't permanently ruin the ride.

I find I still have a need to grieve. Whenever this happens, I stop whatever I'm doing and let myself feel anguish for as long as I need to.

Then I drive on.

Remember to Laugh

Brenda Elsagher and Scott Burton are two comedians who have had cancer and who have used humor as therapy, for themselves and for other people. Another survivor who has written award-winning humorous books is Christine Clifford. She has created the Cancer Club, based near Minneapolis, Minnesota, which serves as an international clearinghouse for people whose lives have been affected by cancer. Christine's books are fun to read, insightful, and filled with wisdom. In her latest book, *Cancer Has Its Privileges,* Christine points out that humor is a great connector of people. She says she found that if she used humor to put people at ease, allowing them to feel more comfortable with her diagnosis, they interpreted her humor as as a sign that she had a positive attitude, and that led to them wanting to surround her with support. (See Resources to find listings for the Cancer Club and for Christine's book.)

Explore the Private Roads of Sexuality

When it comes to sex, it's important to remember that the brain is the primary erogenous zone. The brain is where intimacy starts. It's not uncommon for a person's sexual desire to be diminished during cancer treatments, but the good news is that once your body begins to renew itself, so does your sex drive. If you once had a healthy sexual appetite, having cancer interferes only temporarily with your capacity to fulfill your needs. It may seem that major changes in your body, like an ostomy, would interfere with sexual pleasure. Well, this is one of those areas about which I would say, where there is a will, there is a way. With just a little creativity—and perhaps the alteration of some sexy undergarments—your body can look as good as ever. Using fantasy is also a help when you are struggling with changes in your appearance.

Also, there's nothing like good communication to overcome anxiety about sex, and that's certainly true when it comes to combating negative thoughts caused by problems with your health. A loving sexual partner can help you to regain your perspective.

If you are a woman and have experienced some sexual changes after radiation, such as discomfort during intercourse or vaginal dryness, consult a doctor or a nurse for medical advice. Vaginal dilators, lubricating creams, and frequent intercourse may prove helpful. If you are a man, this time you might really want to ask for directions. Orgasms can occur without ejaculation. For both women and men, two booklets are available: *Sexuality and Cancer*, from the American Cancer Society, and *Sex for the Male/Female Ostomate*, from the United Ostomy Association. (See Resources.)

Finding Meaning after Cancer

Jane Nielsen, in the Winter 2003 issue of the ACE newsletter, *The Advocate*, eloquently sums up what so many of us have learned as cancer survivors:

> There is a small dish on my dressing table that holds five smooth stones. Each is engraved with one word: courage, abundance, freedom, insight, and destiny. The stones were an unexpected find in a gift shop years ago, and their meaning grows with time. They serve as a metaphor for my life journey. Each represents a moment of clarity.

Courage. I recall the courage it took as a scrubbed cancer patient, stripped of my identity, to enter the surgical suite and an uncertain future.

Abundance. The meaning of abundance changed from the right numbers in my checkbook to the right numbers in my lab report.

Freedom. The concept of freedom was reframed as well. Without good health, I am not free to pursue my dreams or to complete what I have begun.

Insight. Insight gained from face-to-face combat with a lethal terrorist—cancer—changed the course of my life and illuminated the way towards purposeful, authentic living.

Destiny. Viewing time as currency, it is my destiny to invest wisely.

❡ ❡ ❡

Along those lines, I'd like to add one more thought to Jane's comments. Morrie Schwartz, in the book *Letting Go,* is quoted as saying, "Take in as much joy as you can whenever and however you can. You may find it in unpredictable places and situations."

I have joined two cancer survivor groups in the last two years. One is ACE (Advocates of Colorectal Education), several of whose members you've met in the pages of this book. The other is the Minneapolis division of the United Ostomy Association. Both of these organizations have helped satisfy my need to give back the kindnesses and support I received during my cancer experience. If you or someone you love is facing this disease, call us, e-mail us, or drop us a letter. The addresses of both of these organizations can be found in the back of the book.

The cancer survivors whose stories appear in these pages have faced cancer head-on. We were amazed to find that the joy in our lives did not go away, nor did our love for our families and friends diminish. Through our struggles we found the best ways to cope with colorectal cancer and, in the process, the best ways to live life to its fullest. We never expected to come out of this experience with such fortitude. We gain a sense of purpose by reaching out to others and helping them cope with colorectal cancer. We will do everything we can to make this an easier journey for you. We promise.

Positive Options after Surviving Cancer

◆ Keep your time balanced between the demands of work and other aspects of your life that are important to you.

◆ Seek the most positive solutions to your problems.

◆ Practice good nutrition. No diet is magic or can "cure" you of your cancer, but a healthy diet with plenty of fruits, vegetables, whole grains, and lean protein is essential for optimizing your well-being. Consult your doctor about taking supplements.

◆ Give support to others as a way to thank the people who have helped you along the way. Encourage others to be screened for colorectal cancer.

◆ Celebrate life. Drive to your favorite park. Smell the roses. Or, if it's fall, go on a hayride. Buy yourself a hot fudge malt. Spend time with the people you love. Sing. Listen to music. Laugh. Have a glass of wine. Enjoy the sunsets.

◆ Hug your children. Or your grandchildren. Or any child. Be thankful.

References

Citations from Books

Burton, Scott, Marnie D. Kenney, and Patrick O'Leary. *A Life in the Balance: A Professional Juggler and Comic's Story of Surviving Cancer with Laughter and a Passion for Living*. Minneapolis, MN: Inconvenience Publications, 1997.

Christiano, Alene, Ed.D. *Radiation and Chemotherapy for Cancer: Mind-Body Therapy for Healing*. Bloomington, IN: First Books Library, 2003, p. 43.

Clifford, Christine. *Cancer Has Its Privileges: Stories of Hope and Laughter*. New York: The Berkley Publishing Group, 2002, p. 24.

Elsagher, Brenda. *If the Battle Is Over, Why Am I Still in Uniform? Humor as a Survival Tactic to Combat Cancer*. Andover, MN: Expert Publishing Inc., 2003, pp. 22, 26, 33, 132, 137–39.

Schwartz, Morrie. *Letting Go*. New York: Delta Publishing, 1997, p. 68.

Excerpts from Articles

The Advocate newsletter, "Survivor Stories," written by ACE members, all issues, 2002–2004; and excerpt from "Finding Meaning," by Jane Nielsen, Winter 2003. (P.O. 14266, St. Paul MN 55114).

Elsagher, Brenda, interview with Marcia Engleson, *Ostomy Outlook*, newsletter of Minneapolis chapter of the United Ostomy Association, #101, May 2002.

Larson, Carol, excerpts from "Lessons Learned from Surviving Cancer," *Coping with Cancer*, Nov./Dec. 2001, p. 55. (P.O. Box 682268, Franklin TN 37068).

Larson, Carol, excerpts from "The Road to Recovery," *Stressfree Living*, Sept. 2003, p. 16. (17483 Sunset Tr., Suite A, Prior Lake MN 55372).

Resources

Online Resources

Alternative cancer therapies, "frequently asked questions": **www.curezone.com**

American Cancer Society, "All about Colon and Rectum Cancer": **www.cancer.org**

American Gastroenterological Association: **www.gastro.org**

Association of Cancer Online Resources: **www.acor.org**

Cancer Research and Prevention Foundation: **www.preventcancer.org**

Choices in Healing: A Guide to Complementary Therapies (operated by the UVA Cancer Center): **www.med.virginia.edu**

Colon Cancer Alliance: **www.ccalliance.org**

Find a colorectal surgeon: **www.fascrs.org**

Find a genetic counselor: **www.nsgc.org/resourcelink.asp**

Frankly speaking about colorectal cancer: **www.thewellnesscommunity.org**

Mayo Foundation for Medical Education and Research: **www.mayo.edu**

Medicare and Medicaid: **www.ssa.gov**

Minnesota Colorectal Cancer Consortium: **www.cancer.umn.edu/coloncanceraware**

National Cancer Institute, click on colon and rectal cancer on the home page: **www.cancer.gov**

Questionable cancer therapies (operated by Stephen Barrett, M.D., and Victor Herbert, M.D., J.D.): **www.quackwatch.com**

Radiation Proctitis: **www.endowsec.com**

United Ostomy Association: **www.uoa.org**

Women's Cancer Network, colorectal cancer information: **www.wcn.org**

Books

On Colorectal Cancer, Cancer in General, and Living with an Ostomy

Bruning, Nancy. *Coping with Chemotherapy.* New York: Avery, 2002.

Bub, David S., M.D., Susannah Rose Rode, MSSW, and W. Douglas Wong, M.D. *100 Questions and Answers about Colorectal Cancer.* Sudbury, MA: Jones and Bartlett Publishers, 2003.

Daniel, Rosy, M.D., with Rachel Ellis. *The Cancer Prevention Book.* Alameda, CA: Hunter House, 2002.

Halvorson-Boyd, Glenna, and Lisa K. Hunter. *Dancing in Limbo.* San Francisco, CA: Jossey-Bass, 1995.

Johnston, Lorraine. *Colon and Rectal Cancer: A Comprehensive Guide for Patients and Families.* Sebastopol, CA: Patient-Centered Guides, a subsidiary of O'Reilly and Associates, 2000.

Kupfer, Barbara, Kathy Foley-Bolch, Michelle Fallon Kasouf, and W. Brian Sweeney, M.D. *Yes We Can! Advice on Traveling with an Ostomy and Tips for Everyday Living.* Worcester, MA: Chandler House Press Books, 2000.

Larson, Carol. *When the Trip Changes: A Traveler's Advisory to Colorectal Cancer.* Minneapolis, MN: Fresh Color Press and Donn Poll Publishing, 2003.

Pazdur, Richard, M.D., and Melanie Royce, M.D. *Myths and Facts about Colorectal Cancers: What You Need to Know.* Huntington, NY: PRR, Inc., 1998.

Weihofen, Donna L., R.D., M.S., with Christina Marino, M.D., MPH. *The Cancer Survival Cookbook.* New York: John Wiley and Sons, 1998.

White, Craig A. *Positive Options for Living with Your Ostomy.* Alameda, CA: Hunter House, 2002.

On Handling Stress

Cameron, Julia. *Blessings.* New York: Penguin Putnam, 1998.

Chopra, Deepak, M.D. *Ageless Body, Timeless Mind.* New York: Harmony Books, 1993.

Helpful Magazines

Coping with Cancer
P. O. Box 682268, Franklin TN 37068
To subscribe, call (615) 791-3859

Cure
3535 Worth St., Colins Tower, Suite 185, Dallas TX 75246
For a free subscription go to www.curetoday.com/freesubscriptions/index.html

Ostomy Quarterly
19772 MacArthur Blvd., Suite 200, Irvine CA 92612
Subscription is free if you join the United Ostomy Association or can be ordered by calling (800) 826-0826.

Stressfree Living
17483 Sunset Trail, Suite A, Prior Lake MN 55372
To subscribe, call (952) 226-5384.

Magazine and Journal Articles

"Focus on Colorectal Cancer." *Coping with Cancer*, March/April 2004, pp. 32–37. (P.O. Box 682268, Franklin TN 37068)

Turnbull, Gwen B., R.N. "Intimacy after Colorectal Surgery." *Ostomy Quarterly*, Winter 2003, pp. 64–65. (19772 MacArthur Blvd., Suite 200, Irvine CA 92612-2405)

Wilcox, S., and M. L. Stefanick. "Knowledge and Perceived Risk of Major Diseases in Middle-Aged and Older Women." *Health Psychology*, vol. 18, 1999, pp. 346–53.

Zangwill, Monica, M.D. "Closing In on Colon Cancer." *Cure*, Spring 2004, pp. 42–49. (Sammons Cancer Center, 3535 Worth St., Suite 4802, Dallas TX 75246-9930)

Useful Organizations

ACE-*Minnesota*
P. O. Box 14266
St. Paul MN 55114   (651) 312-1556
Website: www.acemn.org
Advocates for Colorectal Education (ACE) is a survivor group striving to reduce the incidence of colorectal disease and mortality by advocating

for early education, surveillance, and patient support. (Surveillance involves both screening and being watchful of new ways to combat colorectal cancer.) Offers one-on-one support to patients and caregivers via phone calls, e-mail, or, if possible, personal visits; complimentary "care packets" for patients diagnosed with colorectal cancer; and help in facilitating new groups. For a free copy of their newsletter, which is also free to members, write to the address above or go to ACE's website.

American Cancer Society
1599 Clifton Rd. NE
Atlanta GA 30329-4251   (800) ACS-2345 (800-227-2345)
Website: www.cancer.org
Offers information on colorectal cancer; access to cancer survivors and families through online chats, message boards, and support groups; as well as tips on healthy eating, nutrition information, and recipes. Publishes the helpful pamphlets *Guide to Complementary and Alternative Cancer Methods* and *Sexuality and Cancer.*

The United Ostomy Association, Inc.
19772 MacArthur Blvd., Suite 200
Irvine CA 92612-2405
(800) 826-0826   (949) 660-8624
E-mail: info@uoa.org   Website: www.uoa.org
A volunteer-based health organization that provides support and information regarding ostomy care. Publishes the *Ostomy Quarterly.* Sponsors a yearly conference for members and supports local chapters throughout the United States.

Cancer Information Service, National Cancer Institute
(800) 4-CANCER (800-422-6237)
(800) 332-8615, TTY
Website: www.cancer.gov
Maintains a list of health professionals who specialize in genetics and provide information and counseling. Also a source for locating a colorectal surgeon.

Cancer Research and Prevention Foundation
1600 Duke St., Suite 500
Alexandria VA 22314   (800) 227-2732
(703) 836-4412   (703) 836-4413, fax
E-mail: info@preventcancer.org
Website: www.preventcancer.org

A national, nonprofit health foundation dedicated to the prevention and early detection of cancer through scientific research and education.

R.A. Bloch Foundation
4400 Main St.
Kansas City MO 64111
(800) 433-0464 toll-free national hotline
(816) 932-8453
Cancer survivor Richard Bloch is the founder of the R. A. Bloch Cancer Foundation, which offers free information to cancer patients.

The Cancer Club
6533 Limerick Dr.
Edina MN 55439   (952) 941-1229, fax
E-mail: Christine@cancerclub.com
Acts as an international clearinghouse of information and resources for people affected by cancer and also offers inspirational gifts through a quarterly newsletter. Based in the Minneapolis area, the club was founded by Christine Clifford.

The Colon Cancer Alliance (CCA)
175 Ninth Ave.
New York NY 10011
(877) 422-2030, toll-free helpline   (212) 627-7451, fax
A national patient-advocacy organization dedicated to ending the suffering caused by colorectal cancer. CCA is the official patient-support partner of Katie Couric's National Colorectal Cancer Research Alliance (NCCRA).

Social Security Administration (SSA)
(800) 772-1213
Website: www.ssa.gov
To learn whether you qualify for Social Security Disability Income, Medicare, or Medicaid, contact the SSA and ask for a free booklet to be sent to your address.

Registry Information

Early Detection Research Network High-Risk Registry (EDRN)
The Hereditary Cancer Institute
Creighton University

2500 California Plaza
Omaha NE 68178
(800) 648-8133 x3189
Website: http://medicine2.creighton.edu/EDRN-Regisry
This registry seeks to enroll individuals at high risk for hereditary cancer
and facilitate their participation in early cancer detection research conducted through the network.

Ostomy Supply Retailers

Bruce Medical Supply: **www.brucemedical.com/ostomy**
Duke Medical Supply: **www.dukemedicalsupply.com**
Handi Medical Supply: **www.handimedical.com**
Liberty Medical: **www.LibertyMedical.com**
Medical Supply Group: **www.medicalsupplygroup.com**

Index

POSITIVE OPTIONS FOR CROHN'S DISEASE *by Joan Gomez, M.D.*

Crohn's disease is an inflammatory bowel condition that, while non-fatal, can be devastating. This book discusses who is at risk and why, and addresses what can be done, including self-care.

192 pages ... 1 illus. ... Paperback $12.95

POSITIVE OPTIONS FOR LIVING WITH YOUR OSTOMY
by Dr. Craig A. White

This book is a complete, supportive guide to dealing with the practical and emotional aspects of life after ostomy surgery.

144 pages ... 4 illus. ... Paperback $12.95

POSITIVE OPTIONS FOR HIATUS HERNIA *by Tom Smith, M.D.*

A hiatus hernia is a common, potentially serious condition that occurs when the upper part of the stomach pushes through the diaphragm. This book describes tests, treatments, and self-help options.

128 pages ... 4 illus. ... 2 tables ... Paperback $12.95

POSITIVE OPTIONS FOR COLORECTAL CANCER
by Carol Ann Larson

Colorectal cancer, the second leading cancer killer of adults in the U.S, is treatable if caught in time. This book tells you everything you need to know about prevention, diagnosis, and treatment.

168 pages ... 10 illus. ... Paperback $12.95

**POSITIVE OPTIONS FOR REFLEX SYMPATHETIC DYSTROPHY
(RSD)** *by Elena Juris*

RSD, also called Complex Regional Pain Syndrome, is characterized by severe nerve pain and extreme sensitivity to touch. This book covers medical information, practical advice, and holistic therapies.

224 pages ... 2 illus. ... Paperback $14.95

POSITIVE OPTIONS FOR ANTIPHOSPHOLIPID SYNDROME (APS)
by Triona Holden

Also called Hughes syndrome and "sticky blood," APS is implicated in many serious health problems. This book identifies the symptoms and provides important information on diagnosis and treatment.

144 pages ... Paperback $12.95

POSITIVE OPTIONS FOR SEASONAL AFFECTIVE DISORDER (SAD)
by Fiona Marshall and Peter Cheevers

About 10 million Americans suffer from SAD. This book helps distinguish the condition from classic depression and chronic fatigue, and suggests ways to alleviate the symptoms and live optimally.

144 pages ... Paperback $12.95

All prices subject to change

WOMEN'S CANCERS: How to Prevent Them, How to Treat Them, How to Beat Them — *Third edition*

by Kerry A. McGinn, R.N., and Pamela J. Haylock, R.N.

This guide gives detailed information on treating and surviving the cancers that exclusively affect women: breast, cervical, ovarian, uterine, and vaginal cancer. The second edition also covered lung and colon cancer, as well as the latest screening guidelines and diagnostic tests. The third edition addresses late and long-term effects of cancer, the new FDA approved and "smart" drugs, and possible environmental factors in cancer development.

544 pages ... 72 illus. ... Paperback $24.95

MEN'S CANCERS: How to Prevent Them, How to Treat Them, How to Beat Them ... *Pamela J. Haylock R.N., M.A., E.T., Editor*

This is a resource for men concerned about cancer, their family members, and caregivers. Each chapter is written by a specialized nurse or nurse practitioner and covers prevention, early detection, diagnosis, treatments, follow-up, and recurrence. Special chapters address sex changes related to cancer and future directions in scientific research and study. Includes an extensive resource section.

368 pages ... 16 illus. ... Paperback $19.95

CANCER DOESN'T HAVE TO HURT: How to Conquer the Pain Caused by Cancer and Cancer Treatment

by Pamela J. Haylock, R.N., and Carol P. Curtiss, R.N.

People with cancer often suffer pain needlessly. Research shows that cancer patients who have less pain do better. Readers learn how to describe pain in terms doctors understand and ask for the pain relief they need. The authors explain how to read prescriptions, administer medications, and adjust dosages if necessary. The book also includes information on proven non-drug methods of pain relief.

192 pages ... 10 illus. ... Paperback $14.95

THE PROSTATE HEALTH WORKBOOK: A Practical Guide for the Prostate Cancer Patient *by Newton Malerman, Foreword by Rachmel Cherner, M.D.*

Malerman, a prostate cancer survivor, attributes his recovery to a proactive approach. He encourages readers to understand their disease and get the best medical care possible. Based on his experience, extensive research, and discussions with doctors, nurses, and patients, he has written this hands-on book that includes 25 worksheets, from medical history checklists and treatment evaluation charts to test result records.

160 pages ... 8 illus. 25 worksheets ... Paperback $14.95